Tackling Noncommunicable Diseases in Bangladesh

DIRECTIONS IN DEVELOPMENT
Human Development

Tackling Noncommunicable Diseases in Bangladesh

Now Is the Time

Sameh El-Saharty, Karar Zunaid Ahsan, Tracey L. P. Koehlmoos, and Michael M. Engelgau

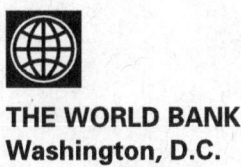

THE WORLD BANK
Washington, D.C.

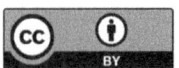

Contents

Preface   *ix*
Acknowledgments   *xi*
About the Authors   *xiii*
Abbreviations   *xvii*

Overview   1
    The Growing Burden of Noncommunicable Diseases in
      Bangladesh   1
    Health System and NCD Capacity   4
    Health Policies, Activities, and Challenges   5
    Key Policy Options and Strategic Priorities   7
    Note   13
    References   13

Chapter 1   **Contexts and Transitions**   17
    Global, Regional, and Country Contexts   17
    Demographic and Epidemiological Transitions   22
    Note   25
    References   25

Chapter 2   **Burden of Disease and Risk Factors for NCDs**   27
    Global and Regional Burden of NCDs   27
    Bangladesh NCD Burden   30
    NCD Risk Factors   38
    Economic and Social Impact   49
    Notes   53
    References   53

Chapter 3   **Health System and NCD Capacity Assessment**   61
    Introduction   61
    Health Service Delivery   61
    Health Workforce   67
    Health Information Systems   69
    Pharmaceuticals and Medical Technology   70
    Health Financing   70

	Health Sector Governance	72
	Note	74
	References	74

Chapter 4	National NCD Activities and Challenges	77
	Orientation of the Public Sector	77
	Country Activities	79
	Challenges	82
	References	85

Chapter 5	Key Policy Options and Strategic Priorities	87
	Stewardship and Regulatory Policy Options and Strategies	88
	Population-Based Policy Options and Strategies for the Non-Health Sector	93
	Population-Based Policy Options and Strategies for the Health Sector	98
	Policy Options and Strategies for Individual Clinical Interventions for the Prevention of NCDs in the Health Sector	99
	Policy Options and Strategies for Individual Clinical Interventions for the Treatment of NCDs in the Health Sector	101
	Lead Role of the Ministry of Health and Family Welfare	103
	References	104

| Appendix 1 | Leading Causes of Mortality and Disability-Adjusted Life Years and Risk Factors for Bangladesh, 2010 Estimates | 107 |

| Appendix 2 | NCD Treatment, Research, and Training Institutions in Bangladesh | 109 |

| Appendix 3 | Assessment and the Program Management Cycle | 115 |

Boxes

1.1	Chapter One Summary	18
2.1	Chapter Two Summary	28
2.2	Methods to Describe the Health Situation in South Asia	29
2.3	Arsenic—Still a Major Public Health Threat	49
3.1	Chapter Three Summary	62
4.1	Chapter Four Summary	78
4.2	Strategic Plan for Surveillance and Prevention of NCDs in Bangladesh, 2011–15	80
5.1	Chapter Five Summary	88
5.2	"Sin Tax" Reform in the Philippines	96

Figures

O.1 A Policy Options Framework for the Prevention and Control
of NCDs 8
1.1 Population in the 21st Century, Bangladesh 22
1.2 Changing Age Structure of the Population in Bangladesh, 2001,
2026, and 2051 23
1.3 Projected Impact of Population Growth and Aging on Total
Health Expenditure in the South Asia Region, 2000–20 23
1.4 NCD Mortality Increases in Rural Bangladesh (Matlab),
1986–2006 24
2.1 Main Causes of Global DALYs and Top Five Risk Factors for
Poor Health, 1990 and 2010 28
2.2 BOD as a Proportion of Total Forgone DALYs by Cause,
Global and South Asia, 2010 29
2.3 Proportion of Total Deaths and Forgone DALYs Due to NCDs,
South Asia, 2004 30
2.4 Leading Causes of Mortality and Morbidity in Bangladesh, 2010
Estimates 31
2.5 Leading Causes of Premature Deaths in Bangladesh, 2010
Estimates 32
2.6 Causes of Deaths among Women of Reproductive Age
(15–49 Years), Bangladesh, 2010 33
2.7 Causes of Mortality among Women of Reproductive Age in
Bangladesh, 2001 and 2010 35
2.8 Distribution of People Who Suffered from Asthma/Respiratory
Diseases in the Preceding 12 Months by Locality,
Bangladesh, 2005 and 2010 36
2.9 Death Rate in Each Age Group from the Five Leading Injury
Causes among Children 37
2.10 Diabetes Prevalence (Self-Reported) among Adults, Aged
25 Years and Above, by Locality and Gender, Bangladesh, 2010 39
2.11 Leading Risk Factors for Bangladesh, 2010 Estimates 40
2.12 Tobacco Use among Adults, Aged 25 Years and Above, by Locality,
Bangladesh, 2010 41
2.13 Prevalence of High Blood Pressure/Hypertension
(BP ≥ 140/90 mmHg or on Medication) among Adults Aged
25 Years or More by Locality and Gender, Bangladesh, 2010 44
2.14 Low Birth Weight and the Transgenerational Effect in Increasing
the Risk of NCDs 45
2.15 Overweight and Obesity Status among Males and Females,
Bangladesh, 2011 47
2.16 Prevalence of Physical Inactivity in Four Sites in Bangladesh 48
2.17 The Macroeconomic Effects of NCDs 50
2.18 Social Determinants, NCDs, and Their Relationship to Poverty 51

3.1   Building Blocks of a Health System   63
3.2   Structure of the Health Service Delivery System in the
       MOHFW   64
3.3   Types of Health Care Providers in Bangladesh, 2007   68
3.4   Share of Public Health Expenditure in Total Health Expenditure
       and in Total Public Expenditure   71
3.5   Bangladesh Governance Indicators, 2000–09   73

Tables

1.1   Demographic, Economic, and Health Profiles for South Asian
       Countries, 2011   19
2.1   Diabetes Prevalence among Urban Men and Women, Aged
       35 Years and Above, by Background Characteristics,
       Bangladesh, 2006   39
2.2   Per Capita Edible Oil Consumption in Bangladesh   43
5.1·   Policy Options Framework for Prevention and Control of NCDs
       in Bangladesh   89
5.2   Estimated Cost of Interventions to Reduce NCD Risk Factors in
       Three Countries   92
5.3   Effects of Salt-Intake Reduction and Tobacco Control
       Interventions in Bangladesh, 2006–15   93
5.4   Role of the Different Sectors in the Prevention and Control
       of NCDs   94
5.5   Recommended Services at Various Levels of Care in the
       MOHFW in Bangladesh   102

Preface

Bangladesh is undergoing rapid demographic and epidemiological transitions, with an increasing older population and a shifting disease burden from infectious, communicable diseases to chronic, noncommunicable diseases (NCDs). The majority of deaths in the country are attributable to NCDs and chronic health conditions. The South Asia Region (SAR) as a whole is experiencing a similar trend, hence the prevention and control of NCDs constitute a priority development issue for low-income countries in SAR, including Bangladesh.

In 2011, a regional report on NCDs in South Asia was published by the World Bank titled *Capitalizing on the Demographic Transition: Tackling Noncommunicable Diseases in South Asia*. It provided a rationale for public policy and action for NCDs in the SAR countries, including Bangladesh, and presented a framework to guide the formulation of public policies and strategies for NCDs from a regional perspective. This current report is built primarily on that regional report, with the goal of stimulating policy dialogue about Bangladesh's health transition and its policy options.

The main objectives of this report are, for Bangladesh:

- To develop an NCD burden and risk factor profile,
- To assess the health system's capacity to prevent and control NCDs,
- To take stock of ongoing NCD activities and identify remaining challenges, and
- To develop a range of policy options and strategies for the prevention and control of NCDs.

The target readership comprises policy makers in the government, both inside and outside the Ministry of Health and Family Welfare, and the program managers in the ministry. The report will also be beneficial for professionals working in the development sector, including partners. The key areas in the Policy Options Framework for Prevention and Control of NCDs (figure O.1) outlined in this report are expected to be instrumental in fostering further intra- and intersectoral collaboration.

This report is organized in such a way that the key policy options and strategic priorities are based on the country context, including the burden of NCDs and associated risk factors and the existing capacity of the health system. Chapter 1 describes the country and regional contexts and the evidence of the demographic and epidemiological transitions in Bangladesh; chapter 2 outlines the disease burden of major NCDs, including the equity and economic impact and the common risk factors; chapter 3 provides an assessment of the health system and its capacity to prevent and control major NCDs; chapter 4 summarizes ongoing NCD interventions/activities in Bangladesh and highlights the remaining gaps and challenges; and chapter 5 presents key policy options and strategic priorities to prevent and control NCDs.

Acknowledgments

This report was prepared by a core team consisting of Sameh El-Saharty, Senior Health Policy Specialist and Team Leader, South Asia Region, the World Bank, Washington, DC, United States; Karar Zunaid Ahsan, Senior Research Associate, MEASURE Evaluation, University of North Carolina at Chapel Hill, NC, Tracey L. P. Koehlmoos, Adjunct Professor, Department of Health Administration and Policy, George Mason University, VA, and Michael Maurice Engelgau, former Senior Health Specialist, South Asia Region, the World Bank, Washington, DC.

The team would like to thank the officials of the Ministry of Health and Family Welfare, Government of Bangladesh, for reviewing the report and providing useful comments and feedback, including: Dr. Khondhaker Md. Shefayatullah, Director General, Directorate General of Health Services (DGHS), and Line Director, Noncommunicable Disease Control (NCDC); Dr. AKM Jafarullah, Deputy Program Manager, NCD & Arsenic, NCDC, DGHS; Prof. Mahmudur Rahman, Director, Institute of Epidemiology, Disease Control and Research, DGHS; and Dr. MA Faiz, Professor of Medicine, Sir Salimullah Medical College. Dr. M Mostafa Zaman, National Professional Officer (Noncommunicable Diseases), World Health Organization, Bangladesh also provided resources and useful information.

The team is grateful to the peer reviewers of the report for their constructive comments. The peer reviewers from Bangladesh are: Prof. Dr. Shah Monir Hossain, former Director General of the DGHS; Prof. Dr. Md. Habibe Millat, Vice Chairman and Honorary Director, Bangladesh Medical Research Council, Bangladesh; and Associate Professor Dr. Sohel Reza Choudhury, Project Coordinator, Anti Tobacco Program, Department of Epidemiology and Research, National Heart Foundation Hospital and Research Institute, Bangladesh. The peer reviewers from the World Bank are Patricio Marquez, Lead Health Specialist, Africa Region; Anne Maryse Pierre-Louis, Lead Public Health Specialist, the Health, Nutrition, and Population Network; Montserrat Meiro-Lorenzo, Senior Public Health Specialist, the Health, Nutrition and Population Network; and Shiyong Wang, Senior Health Specialist, Middle East and North Africa Region.

The team would like to thank several World Bank colleagues who provided comments on different drafts of this report including Andras Horvai, Country Program Coordinator, Bangladesh Country Team; and Albertus Voetberg, Lead

Health Specialist, Bushra Binte Alam, Senior Health Specialist, Nkosinathi Mbuya, Senior Nutrition Specialist, and Iffat Mahmud, Operations Officer, Human Development, South Asia Region.

Special thanks go to Mashida Rashid and Shahela Anwar, Research Assistants, ICDDR,B. Operational support was provided by Alejandro Welch, the World Bank. Assistance in editing the report was provided by Jonathan Aspin (consultant).

Finally, the core team would like to extend its gratitude to Julie McLaughlin, Health, Nutrition, and Population Sector Manager, and Jesko Hentschel, Human Development Director, both in the South Asia Region, the World Bank, for their guidance and support during the preparation of the study and the dissemination of the final report.

About the Authors

Sameh El-Saharty MD, MSc, MPH, works as Senior Health Policy Specialist in the South Asia region at the World Bank in Washington, DC. He is responsible for leading the preparation and implementation of large projects in the region, coordinating the regional reproductive health program, coordinating the work of the Asia Pacific Observatory on health policy and systems research in the region, and leading several projects to provide technical and advisory work. Before joining the Bank, he held several positions with international organizations, academic institutions, and consulting firms such as U.S. Agency for International Development, United Nations Population Fund, Harvard University, the American University in Cairo, and Pathfinder International. He has over 28 years' experience working as a researcher, technical adviser and international consultant on public health, health policy and management, health insurance, and health sector reform programs in more than 18 countries in the Middle East and North Africa region, Africa, South Asia, and in the United States.

He authored and contributed to more than 30 published articles, policy notes, strategy papers, technical studies, analytical reports, and books. His recent work has focused on health systems with particular interest in health service delivery. His most recent work includes two World Bank publications entitled *Capitalizing on the Demographic Transition: Tackling Noncommunicable Diseases in South Asia* and *Improving Health Service Delivery in Developing Countries: From Evidence to Action.* He has been a guest speaker and lecturer in different academic and research institutions.

He is currently a member of the Harvard School of Public Health (HSPH) Dean's Leadership Council, HSPH Alumni Council, and the Advisory Committee of the MENA Health Policy Forum. He is a licensed medical doctor graduated from Cairo University and holds a Master of Sciences in Public Health from the Military Medical Academy in Egypt, and a Master of Public Health from Harvard University.

Karar Zunaid Ahsan has worked in the fields of monitoring, evaluation, and research in the health sector for over 10 years, most recently as a Senior M & E Resident Advisor for Bangladesh at MEASURE Evaluation to carry out M & E, research, survey, and capacity building in Bangladesh's Health, Nutrition, and Population (HNP) sector program. Before working at MEASURE, he worked for four years for the World Bank's South Asia Human Development Sector as a research analyst where he was involved with developing knowledge products and strategic analytical tasks in Bangladesh's HNP sector.

He has authored 18 reports and book chapters and had 6 articles published in peer-reviewed journals. He has also presented in various international symposiums and conferences on issues related to care-seeking behavior, health systems strengthening, epidemiologic and demographic transitions, and population projections.

He graduated in Applied Statistics (Econometrics) from the University of Dhaka and completed a Master of International Public Health from the University of Sydney.

Dr. Tracey Pérez Koehlmoos PhD, MHA, is the Special Assistant to the Assistant Commandant of the United States Marine Crops. Previously, she served as the Programme Head for Health and Family Planning Systems at ICDDR,B in Dhaka, Bangladesh. She specializes in health systems research ranging from upstream activities such as improving service delivery in hard-to-reach areas and the urban homeless and demand-side financing, to more downstream areas to include the translation of evidence to policy and national scaling up of zinc. She founded the Centre for Systematic Review at ICDDR,B, which specializes in reviews of health policy and systems issues in the nonstate sector. She developed the Centre for Control of Chronic Diseases in Bangladesh, which includes expansive research, education, and knowledge translation components.

She is an adjunct professor in the James P. Grant School of Public Health, BRAC University, and in the College of Health and Human Services, George Mason University. She serves on the Cochrane Library Oversight Committee and on the advisory board of the International Development Coordinating Group of the Campbell Collaboration and has built capacity for systematic reviews across South Asia.

She has lived and worked in South and Southeast Asia for most of her adult life and served as a consultant to the Institute of Medicine, World Health Organization, the World Bank, and the World Food Programme. Her publications appear in the *Cochrane Database of Systematic Reviews, BMJ, The Lancet, PLoS Medicine,* and *Health Research Policy & Systems.*

Michael Engelgau MD, MS, is the Director for China NCD Activities with the U.S. Centers for Disease Control and Prevention (CDC). He has been assigned to the U.S. CDC office in Beijing, China, since June 2011, where he manages the portfolios for noncommunicable disease research and capacity building.

Before this position he completed a four-year assignment with the World Bank (2007–11), during which he was the lead consultant for the Bank's noncommunicable disease portfolio and led several studies on noncommunicable diseases in South Asia. His most recent work is *Capitalizing on the Demographic Transition: Tackling Noncommunicable Diseases in South Asia,* published in June 2011. Prior to the World Bank assignment, he was with the CDC's Division of Diabetes

Translation from 1992, where he held several key positions, including the Division's Directorship in 2006.

During his time with the World Bank and CDC, his focus has been on research programs and policies that translate science into practice to prevent and control noncommunicable diseases. He has been extensively published in peer-reviewed U.S. and international scientific literature with over 190 manuscripts, letters, reports, and book chapters.

After earning his BA and MS at Oregon State University, he obtained his MD at Oregon Health Science University. He completed residencies in both internal medicine and preventive medicine and training with CDC's Epidemic Intelligence Service. He is board certified with the American Board of Internal Medicine and is a Fellow of the American College of Physicians.

Abbreviations

ACE	angiotensin converting enzyme
BADAS	Diabetic Association of Bangladesh
BanNet	Bangladesh Network for Non-Communicable Disease Surveillance and Prevention
BBS	Bangladesh Bureau of Statistics
BIRDEM	Bangladesh Institute of Research and Rehabilitation in Diabetes, Endocrine and Metabolic Disorders
BMI	body mass index
BMMS	Bangladesh Maternal Mortality and Health Care Survey
BOD	burden of disease
BP	blood pressure
BRAC	Bangladesh Rural Advancement Committee
CHD	coronary heart disease
CIPRB	Centre for Injury Prevention and Research, Bangladesh
COPD	chronic obstructive pulmonary disease
CVD	cardiovascular disease
DALY	disability-adjusted life year
DGFP	Directorate General of Family Planning
DGHS	Directorate General of Health Services
GDP	gross domestic product
GNI	gross national income
HIES	Household Income and Expenditure Survey
HPNSDP	Bangladesh Health, Population and Nutrition Sector Development Programme
ICDDR,B	International Centre for Diarrhoeal Disease Research, Bangladesh
IDF	International Diabetes Federation
IEDCR	Institute of Epidemiology, Disease Control and Research
IFG	impaired fasting glucose
IGT	impaired glucose tolerance

IHP	Institute for Health Policy
MDG	Millennium Development Goal
MIS	Management Information System
MMR	maternal mortality ratio
MOHFW	Ministry of Health and Family Welfare
MRC	(British) Medical Research Council
NCCRFHD	National Centre for Control of Rheumatic Fever and Heart Diseases
NCD	noncommunicable disease
NCDC	Non-Communicable Disease Control
NGO	nongovernmental organization
NHFH&RI	National Heart Foundation Hospital and Research Institute
NICRH	National Institute of Cancer Research & Hospital
NICVD	National Institute of Cardiovascular Diseases
NIDCH	National Institute of Diseases & Chest & Hospital
NIMHR	National Institute of Mental Health and Research
NIPORT	National Institute of Population Research and Training
NIPSOM	National Institute of Preventive and Social Medicine
OECD	Organisation for Economic Co-operation and Development
PHC	primary health care
R&D	research and development
SVRS	Sample Vital Registration System
TASC	Alliance of Safe Children
TFR	total fertility rate
WHO	World Health Organization

All dollar amounts are in U.S. dollars unless otherwise indicated.

Overview

The Growing Burden of Noncommunicable Diseases in Bangladesh

Country Context

Bangladesh faces health challenges from avoidable mortality, persistent poverty, a geographic location prone to natural disasters, inefficiencies in governance, and a fertility rate that remains high (despite improving). In addition, population growth and a changing age structure are coupled with economic and social changes that are affecting health, particularly through noncommunicable diseases (NCDs).

Bangladesh is one of the poorest countries in the world—in 2010, an estimated 32 percent of the population lived below the national poverty line (World Bank 2013). As with other countries in the region, the majority live in rural areas, which adds to the challenges both of addressing the causes of NCDs and of delivering care. Around 28 percent of the population recently lived in urban areas (World Bank 2013), but the country is rapidly urbanizing. Dhaka, the capital, is expected to have a population of 22 million by 2025 (up from 9 million in 2007), placing it among the 10 largest cities in the world (NIPORT et al. 2008). In 2007, an estimated 37 percent of Dhaka's population lived in slums (Islam 2005); more than three-quarters of new migrants to Dhaka move to urban slums or areas with even less shelter (Streatfield and Karar 2008).

Despite periods of political turmoil and frequent natural disasters in Bangladesh, the last decade has been marked by sustained growth, stable macroeconomic management, significant poverty reduction, and rapid social transformation and human development. Since the turn of the century, aggregate gross domestic product (GDP) has been rising at a respectable 5.3 percent a year in real terms, or by 4.0 percent per capita, contributing to a decline in poverty from 49.0 percent in 2000 to 32.0 percent in 2010 (World Bank 2013), in a period when Bangladesh had disproportionate poverty reduction for its growth. There has been a continuous reduction in annual population growth from 2.3 percent in 1981 to 1.2 percent in 2011 (BBS 2012; World Bank 2013). Life expectancy at birth for men and women is rising constantly and stands at 69 years, up from 58 years in 1994 (BBS 2011a; World Bank 2013).

Demographic and Epidemiological Transitions

In spite of the country's turbulent and disadvantaged past, the health status of the population has made tremendous strides in terms of reducing fertility and maternal and child mortality. New population and health challenges come from rapid demographic and epidemiological transitions, urbanization, the emerging burden of NCDs, and vulnerability to climate change.

The proportion of the population aged 60 years or more is projected to increase hugely, such that the elderly will make up 18.8 percent of the total population by mid-century, potentially increasing the NCD burden greatly (Streatfield and Karar 2008). A substantial decline in the proportion of the population under 15 years and of females of reproductive age is expected over the next 50 years (El-Saharty et al. forthcoming). Such demographic changes will have a serious impact on health expenditures. An overall rise of about 47.7 percent in health spending between 2000 and 2020 is projected, due to population growth (29.7 percent) and aging (about 18.0 percent), exacerbated by growth in NCDs (Gottret and Schieber 2010).

Burden of Disease and Risk Factors for NCDs

In South Asian countries, the burden of disease (BOD) is shifting—NCDs (including injuries) now account for a larger proportion of forgone disability-adjusted life years than communicable diseases, maternal and child health issues, and nutrition causes combined (59 versus 42 percent) (WHO 2008). This pattern is similar to that of high-income countries decades ago.

A study of 52 countries including Bangladesh found that in South Asia, people suffering their first heart attack were six years younger (at 53 years) than those in the rest of the world, due to high levels of risk factors such as diabetes and high cholesterol, and low levels of protective factors (physical activity and dietary habits). This greater susceptibility to NCDs in South Asia will lead to a bigger disease burden (Goyal and Yusuf 2006; Ramaraj and Chellappa 2008).

Among 23 developing countries studied, Bangladesh ranked ninth in rates of age-standardized mortality due to chronic diseases (Abegunde et al. 2007), primarily cardiovascular diseases (CVDs), and diabetes. Some 68 percent of deaths in Bangladesh are due to NCDs and other chronic health conditions including old age complications (BBS 2011a). A study in medical college hospitals found that about one-third of hospital admissions in patients aged 30 years and over were due to major NCDs (DGHS 2007).[1]

As the burden shifts from surviving birth, childhood, and childbirth, so must the focus of the country's health system shift to continue meeting the needs of the population, particularly the poor. There is no free or subsidized treatment for NCDs through the government health system (unlike for some communicable diseases and maternal and child health programs). Health services are, in principle, free in the public sector, but lack of drugs and indirect costs (for example, transport) result in high out-of-pocket spending by NCD patients.

The major causes of mortality from NCDs are CVDs, cancer, respiratory diseases, injuries, and diabetes (IHME forthcoming). Aside from injuries, all are linked to a few common risk factors—high tobacco use, air pollution (including indoor fires for cooking and heating), poor diet and nutrition, occupational risks, high blood pressure, malnutrition and low birth weight, lack of physical activity, and alcohol consumption and substance abuse. With other social determinants such as poverty, low education, urbanization, and changing lifestyles, the risk of NCDs rises. These factors have long-lasting, transgenerational impacts.

The highlights of the NCD burden and associated risk factors are:

- 7.3 percent of the population have CVDs (BBS 2011b);
- 66 percent of cancer patients are of working age (DGHS 2008);
- The country has some of the highest tobacco use in the world among both men and women (WHO 2011);
- Salt intake is high (Choudhury et al. 2010; WHO 2010);
- The rate of low birth weight (36.0 percent) is among the highest in the world; and (UNICEF/BBS 2005)
- More than 40.0 percent of children under five are either underweight or moderately stunted (NIPORT et al. 2009).

Equity and the Economic Burden

The burden of NCDs varies across socioeconomic strata and gender. For example, the richest households have higher levels of high blood pressure and diabetes (NIPORT et al. 2013), with the greater extremes in slum areas (NIPORT et al. 2008). The prevalence of serious injury among males and females aged 15–59 worsens with decreasing socioeconomic status (NIPORT et al. 2008).

There are few studies of the economic impact of NCDs in Bangladesh. One World Health Organization (WHO) study found that tobacco was a major risk factor and cost the economy about $44 million annually (WHO SEARO 2007). For low-income groups, direct costs associated with diabetic care could drain up to 24.5 percent of annual household income. Expenditures on the risk factors for NCDs (such as tobacco) and the management of these disorders can also adversely affect the financial status of families. Treatment for diabetes can cost 6–12 months' wages ($160 a year). Another study showed that about half of rural poor households in Bangladesh had not been poor before a traffic accident. These findings—alongside high out-of-pocket spending, especially for medication—highlight the need to address financing and equity issues.

Thus the NCD epidemic has a huge direct impact on financial vulnerability, particularly for the poor, and an indirect impact on the economy. Policy makers should consider both these factors when formulating NCD-related policies, aided by considering the social determinants of NCDs as they play an important role in health, and dramatic differences are closely linked to the degree of social disadvantage and poverty within countries.

Health System and NCD Capacity

The prevention and management of NCDs are largely governed by the available capacity of the health system, but assessments of that capacity can be more challenging than for BOD and tend to be less frequent. The assessment here of the overall system's capacity to manage NCDs is considered under seven headings:

- *Health Service Delivery.* The government's role in NCDs is limited to providing health education at primary level and preventive and clinical treatment at tertiary level, with less focus on preventive clinical care at primary and secondary levels, while the private sector provides mainly treatment services. Nongovernmental organizations (NGOs), private providers (formal and informal), and traditional medicine play a large role in service delivery. The National Health Policy 2001 is being updated to ensure that access to health services is pro-poor. A few strategies and guidelines on NCDs exist but there is no good awareness-raising system to keep policy makers abreast of these concerns.

- *Health Workforce.* In 2007, the country had an estimated 7.7 qualified health care providers (BHW 2008) per 10,000 of the population (WHO recommends 25.0 [WHO 2006]), but physicians and nurses account for only 5.0 percent of all health care providers, as most of these are informally trained and cater to the needs of the majority, particularly the poor. Until recently, few health workers were trained in NCD prevention and management but in 2013, the number has increased.

- *Health Information Systems.* Bangladesh has no community public health program or national surveillance for NCDs. Only specialized, tertiary-level hospital-based information is available. Some NCD risk factors are being addressed in Dhaka's population by the National Institute of Preventive and Social Medicine (NIPSOM) and Bangladesh Institute of Research and Rehabilitation in Diabetes, Endocrine and Metabolic Disorders (BIRDEM).

- *Pharmaceuticals.* The pharmaceutical sector is thriving with a national essential drugs policy, but drugs for treating NCDs were only recently included in the list of essential drugs.

- *Health Financing.* Total health expenditure (public and private) accounted for 3.5 percent of GDP in 2011. Per capita health expenditure—inadequate to secure basic services—was about $23 in 2011, a third government financed (Engelgau et al. 2011; World Bank 2013). Although the budget allocated for the NCD line directorate increased to $70 million for 2011–16, this and the portion allocated for NCD awareness are not enough to address the growing NCD challenges, particularly CVDs.

- *Health Sector Governance.* Overall government effectiveness in Bangladesh is weak and has deteriorated significantly since 2000. Accountability and regulatory quality are also low. Tackling NCDs requires an effective governance system to coordinate the multisectoral interventions, a strong regulatory framework to issue new laws and regulations, and increased capacity to enforce them.

Health Policies, Activities, and Challenges

Policies

The public sector program is oriented to primary health care focused on mothers and children as well as communicable disease interventions to meet health-related Millennium Development Goals (MDGs). Four NCDs—CVDs, cancer, diabetes mellitus, and arsenicosis—are identified as major public health concerns. Priorities in the current Strategic Plan for the Health, Population and Nutrition Sector Development Programme (HPNSDP) 2011–16 include expanding NCD control at all levels by streamlining referral systems and strengthening hospital accreditation and management systems. This Strategic Plan recommends that the public sector focus on prevention and that investment in intensive care units and tertiary care be left to the private sector.

Public sector infrastructure is underdeveloped at primary health care level to support NCD prevention and management. NCD program-based infrastructure is largely at tertiary level. There is a long tradition—dating back to the 1950s—of public and nonpublic specialty hospitals and foundations that provide preventive and curative care for NCDs. The HPNSDP Strategic Plan emphasizes the reduction of morbidity and premature mortality due to NCDs in an integrated manner, from primary prevention to treatment and rehabilitation. The operational plans under HPNSDP aim to strengthen health service delivery for effective management and referral, to promote healthy lifestyles and practices, and to develop a sound public health surveillance system.

Activities

Activities on NCDs are mostly carried out through a variety of specialty hospitals and foundations, and participation from the public sector research foundations that play a leading role in national surveillance efforts. Yet despite the aim of the HPNSDP Strategic Plan to include NCD prevention and care at all levels, these activities have been less a priority at the primary care level, which focuses on maternal and child health services and communicable diseases for achieving the MDGs and following the Health for All initiative's emphasis on primary care. The launch of the government's Strategic Plan for Surveillance and Prevention of Noncommunicable Diseases in Bangladesh, 2007–10 and its update in 2011 have, though, helped the country to make great strides toward addressing NCD surveillance and management by the health sector.

NCD activities, public and private, include training and awareness-building workshops; support for the purchase of equipment; expanded NCD health care delivery to district hospitals and selected *upazila* (subdistrict) health complexes through new NCD specialist posts; workshops for community mobilization; community-based surveillance and prevention programs to prevent child injuries; an arsenic mitigation program to raise community awareness, build capacity, and identify patients; a management program to raise awareness of alternate sources of water; research and development and coordination across the public and NGO sectors in arsenic mitigation; expansion by the nonprofit Diabetic Association of Bangladesh of activities to cardiac care and the Health Care Development Program (a model of integrated care service delivery in urban and rural areas with a focus on the major NCDs); restrictions on smoking in public places and tobacco advertising in publications and the mass media; and the aim of the Centre for Control of Chronic Diseases in Bangladesh to bring scientific rigor to the study of the BOD for NCDs, to develop community-based prevention and management programs, to evaluate the link between NCDs and poverty in Bangladesh, and to assess the health system's response to NCDs.

Challenges

The following challenges stand out:

- *The regulatory framework needs to be strengthened.* Improving the regulations that govern the prevention and control of NCDs and their enforcement is critical, including the Smoking and Tobacco Product Usage (Control) Act 2005, which went into effect in May 2006. These, however, require evaluation, and none has yet been conducted. Further, the ban on advertising of tobacco products under the act is incomplete, and smoking is still permitted in a range of areas. Most important, the National Tobacco Control Cell is understaffed and underfunded.

- *Strategic planning and coordination are lacking across sectors.* Several NCD interventions exist in public and private sectors with very little national coordination. There has been no overall assessment of activities by different stakeholders to ensure synergies across these programs, and the focus of the Ministry of Health and Family Welfare (MOHFW) on NCDs remains limited in implementing NCD interventions through the Non-Communicable Disease Control (NCDC) operational plan and financing tertiary health facilities. An evaluation of the Health, Nutrition and Population Sector Programme (2003–11) noted that NCD operational plans were inadequate in leadership, programs, and implementation, despite the priority attached to NCDs in the revised implementation plan in 2008. The government should use its resources to play a leadership role and incorporate NCD prevention and treatment in the public health sector, with support from WHO and already-engaged nonprofit organizations.

- *The objectives and interventions identified in the HPNSDP Strategic Plan are not fully reflected in the operational plans.* For example, the NCDC operational plan primarily focuses on awareness building, but fails to fully pursue training activities of health care providers and to strengthen prevention, detection, and management of major NCDs and/or risk factors in the primary health care system. The Bangladesh Health Workforce Strategy 2008 has not set any specific strategic goal to deal with the workforce to manage NCDs or any activity for implementing the strategic objectives. The Essential Services

Package and the essential drugs list in the public sector do not have guidelines and products to meet the needs of the growing number of individuals at risk for chronic conditions, nor to manage them.

- *The health system focuses on treatment, not prevention.* NCDs are tackled at the secondary and tertiary levels mainly through treatment in specialized facilities. There is less emphasis on prevention at the primary care level and on readily available low-cost treatment. Much of the investment in infrastructure and medical equipment in the specialized facilities could be saved if NCD prevention interventions were scaled up. The Directorate General of Health Services should scale up programs built on an NCD pilot program in *upazilas* under a careful strategy to preserve resources.

- *The health service delivery system is fragmented, leading to lack of coordinated care that is critical for effectively managing NCDs.* In addressing the MDG challenges, the health service delivery system—as in most developing countries— was structured to deal with "episodes" of maternal and child health illnesses and communicable diseases. Shifting the BOD toward NCDs would require an integrated approach that ensures continuity of care.

- *There is an urgent need to fill the data gaps related to NCDs.* The Demographic and Health Surveys and Utilization of Essential Service Delivery Survey focus on fertility, family planning, and maternal and child health but (apart from tobacco use in the former) exclude NCDs. Nor is there a plan to conduct surveillance of NCD morbidity and/or mortality, which would benefit health planning. Finally, rapid urbanization requires a uniform reporting system for urban health care services, enabling the unique risks to the more than 35 percent of slum dwellers in urban areas to be captured and allowing services to be developed for their needs.

Key Policy Options and Strategic Priorities

Tackling NCDs comprehensively would require the adoption of an integrated approach to mobilize the different sectors of the government, as well as the forging of a partnership between the public and private sectors. Figure O.1 represents a Policy Options Framework for the Prevention and Control of NCDs, further elaborated in table 5.1 of the main text.

The framework is founded on the "Stewardship and Regulatory" role that should be led by the health sector, represented by the MOHFW, including mobilizing the non-health sector. This role will serve as the foundation for two broad categories: population-based and individual-based policy interventions, on which four pillars are grounded: multisectoral and health sector interventions, and clinical preventive and treatment services.

Each policy intervention mobilizes different parts of the health and non-health sectors and requires very different inputs in infrastructure, capacity, and

Figure O.1 A Policy Options Framework for the Prevention and Control of NCDs

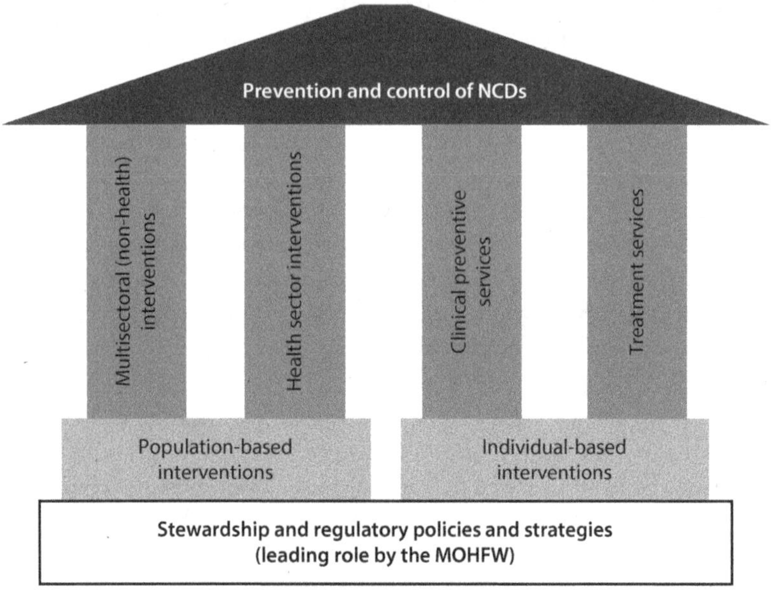

Note: MOHFW = Ministry of Health and Family Welfare; NDC = noncommunicable disease.

skill sets, while yielding very different outputs and outcomes. Harmonizing both sets of policy interventions is necessary to ensure that the mix is right and that population-based policy interventions complement those delivered to individuals within the clinical care system.

A key initial challenge is to determine the strategic priorities that will constitute the steps and capitalize on existing activities, while taking into account the available resources. These strategic priorities should consider the main common risk factors, namely high tobacco use, air pollution, poor diet and nutrition, occupational risks, high blood pressure, malnutrition and low birth weight, lack of physical activity, and alcohol consumption and substance abuse.

The following represents the key highlights of the "options" on policies and strategies to tackle NCDs in Bangladesh. It draws on the above framework and on global best practices taking into consideration the BOD, risk factors, system capacity, and national programs for NCDs in the country. Without being prescriptive, it forms the basis for policy dialog on how to integrate interventions into the national NCD program.

Stewardship and Regulatory Policy Options and Strategies
Representing the health sector, the MOHFW has the leading role in combating NCDs, including mobilizing the non-health sector. The MOHFW will have to spearhead development and implementation of these strategic priorities, which will require their full integration in the relevant operational plans. These steps will also demand new skills so that the MOHFW can work effectively and

lead with other sectors to build a multisectoral alliance to ensure synergy among actions. Further, the MOHFW should consider:

- *Periodically assessing NCD mortality, morbidity, BOD, risk factors, and high-risk populations as well as NCD risk factor determinants in the non-health sector and beyond that the gaps in the policy and regulatory framework for NCD prevention and control.* The MOHFW will need to track utilization, expenditures, institutionalization of activities, and the limits to what surveillance can achieve. Also, it is important to assess the gaps in regulations related to tobacco, commerce, agriculture, trade, the environment, and urban areas. Involving other government sectors and the private sector will be vital (for instance, taxing tobacco by the Ministry of Finance, and lowering carbon emissions by the commerce, industry, and transport sectors).

- *Assessing current and future public health spending and health system capacity (institutional and management capacity and system intelligence) as well as health service delivery capacity (facilities, human resources, drugs, and so on) and current utilization of ambulatory and inpatient care.* A full assessment would cover all health system components including governance, regulatory framework, and institutional capacity; health financing including current and future public health spending and out-of-pocket spending; health service delivery and its infrastructure at all levels as well as its utilization, human resources (numbers and skills), pharmaceuticals and medical technologies, and health system intelligence.

- *Reviewing evidence-based public policies, population-based interventions, and cost-effective prevention and treatment interventions (including in other similar countries).* International experience presents ample evidence on cost-effective interventions such as tobacco control (particularly tobacco taxation), salt reduction, improved diets and physical activity, reduction in hazardous alcohol intake, enforcement of seat belt use, early detection/screening for diabetes and high blood pressure, low-dose aspirin for high-risk CVD patients, and essential drugs and technologies. Priority should be given to population-based interventions given their relatively low cost and greater population benefits, such as using mass media to send positive health messages, particularly to young people. The MOHFW, with help from public or nongovernment research institutes, should explore cost-effective NCD screening programs at community level with a special emphasis on CVDs and/or diabetes. Multidisciplinary research committees should be established in collaboration with academia and professional organizations to look into a sustainable funding mechanism for NCD research; networking of government agencies, NGOs, and the academic community to support research; and translation of research findings to action.

- *Developing a national policy and multisectoral strategic plan for the prevention and treatment of NCDs in consultation with the major stakeholders (health and non-health, public and private) and improving coordination across the NCD program.* Bangladesh does not have a comprehensive national policy and multisectoral strategic plan for NCDs. One should be developed urgently, given the rising NCD epidemic. Several sectors (including the private sector) should be involved in developing the plan, such as finance, agriculture, the food industry, environment, infrastructure, transport, education, media, social protection, the legislature, and law enforcement. Further, the MOHFW will need to take a more active role in coordinating and facilitating the programs that support NCD initiatives in order to build on successful ones and ensure synergies.

Population-Based Policy Options and Strategies for the Non-Health Sector

The government will need to consider the following policy options that would involve the different sectors:

- *Developing and enforcing laws and regulatory mechanisms for the non-health sector.* Several policy actions in the non-health sector can be taken to curb NCDs:
  - *Strengthen tobacco control policies:* The government should consider developing a tax framework that includes all major tobacco products. This could have a great impact on reducing consumption. The experience of the Philippines (box 5.1) in passing a "sin tax" by harnessing political support, engaging different stakeholders, and using evidence-based analytical work may serve as a good example. The government may also consider strictly enforcing other nonprice policy interventions such as banning tobacco-product advertisements and smoking in government premises and public places (such as transport) as a starting point to further expand the ban to larger public areas, as well as pushing through tobacco-supply reductions and information dissemination.
  - *Strengthen food regulation policies:* Studies show that a salt reduction strategy is highly cost effective. The MOHFW should lead a massive public health campaign for reducing salt intake. Similarly, legislation requiring the food industry to substitute 2 percent of transfat with polyunsaturated fat, at $0.50 per adult, is a viable primary intervention for preventing heart disease. The experience of Argentina in reaching agreements with food industry representatives and companies on a progressive and voluntary course to reduce salt in processed foods provides a practical example.
  - *Strengthen control policies on road traffic injuries:* Improving road conditions is critical but will need heavy infrastructure investment. Over a shorter time frame, law enforcement for the use of seat belts and helmets, coupled with a behavior-change campaign, would be feasible and effective to reduce the burden of road traffic accidents.
  - *Develop strategies to reduce child injury:* After infancy, injury is the leading cause of death among children in Bangladesh, accounting for 38 percent of all classifiable deaths. This means that 83 children a day die of injuries. To prevent drowning or road traffic accidents, for example, strategies should

target homes, schools, and the community. Mother and child health clinics can start with awareness building during their regular prenatal checkups and immunizations.

• *Developing the institutional and human capacity of the non-health sector to address NCD risk factor determinants, mobilize the necessary financial resources, and develop an effective monitoring and evaluation system.* Greater institutional capacity is needed to implement regulations and programs. Actions could be supported by allocations of some of the revenues from the tobacco tax to the sectors involved in NCD prevention and control. Professional organizations and civil society can play an important role. In addition, monitoring the results and evaluating the impact of these policies will be key for building the evidence base for future policies.

Population-Based Policy Options and Strategies for the Health Sector

The MOHFW may need to consider the following actions as its primary options:

• *Strengthening the health promotion and risk reduction interventions of the MOHFW for the general population and/or high-risk groups.* This could include promoting more healthy lifestyles and increasing awareness of the risks of smoking, obesity, and respiratory tract infections. Resources should be better used and harmonized. For instance, the Arsenic Control Program is large and commands many resources, which can be used more effectively in more strategic areas like screening and early detection of high blood pressure/hypertension and diabetes.

• *Developing the institutional and human capacity to manage population-based health promotion and risk reduction in the MOHFW, and an effective system intelligence and information technology for NCDs, as well as strengthening and expanding the national surveillance system to include NCDs and their risk factors.* The MOHFW will need to develop the skills of its staff in designing and implementing behavior-change campaigns and health literacy programs to promote healthy lifestyles. Developing an effective system intelligence—that will collect NCD morbidity and mortality data from the service delivery system, monitor trends in risk factors, analyze epidemiological data, and triangulate data from different sources—is becoming increasingly crucial. Much has been done toward a national surveillance system, but an integrated strategy for injury surveillance is needed.

Policy Options and Strategies for Individual Clinical Interventions for Prevention of NCDs in the Health Sector

Along with the options above, the MOHFW will need to adopt, on a priority basis, many of the following actions as complementary to the population-based interventions while engaging the private sector:

• *Developing and implementing basic health services for reducing risk factors and preventing NCDs in public health facilities.* Studies conducted in Bangladesh have demonstrated that diabetic education programs and lifestyle interventions of a nonpharmacological approach can significantly improve self-regulatory behavior, reducing morbidity and mortality related to high blood pressure and diabetes. To ensure effective delivery of a revised Essential Services Package, adequate human resources and infrastructure need to be put in place, such as screening for high blood pressure, cholesterol, and diabetes as well as a communication program for smoking cessation and improved diet.

- *Strengthening the institutional and human resources capacity to provide facility-based health promotion, behavior change, and risk-reduction services.* Beyond expanding the Essential Services Package to include NCD-related interventions is a need for commensurate efforts to strengthen the institutional and human resources capacity to provide these services, particularly those related to integrating primary health care services and to ensuring continuity of care (through training service providers, infrastructure, clinical quality assessment, and provider guidelines).

- *Mobilizing additional financial resources for the health sector, and considering budget reallocation within the health sector in support of NCD prevention and treatment.* The MOHFW will need to engage in a constructive dialogue with the Ministry of Finance and the Prime Minister's Office to mobilize additional resources for the underfinanced health sector, while considering potential efficiency gains. Additional investments in NCDs today will reduce and save future costs that the MOHFW will otherwise have to bear as the result of inaction.

- *Establishing a monitoring system for the NCD prevention indicators in public health facilities as well as conducting impact evaluation studies.* Some process and output indicators may be included in NCD operational plans, commensurate with their funding. In parallel, basic NCD interventions (such as blood pressure and blood glucose measurement for screening, and health promotion) need to be monitored in primary health facilities and included in routine reporting. Data on already-implemented, critical NCD-prevention interventions in tertiary hospitals should also be collected. Data from several other operational plans that support NCD prevention (Health Education and Promotion; Quality Assurance; and Information, Education and Communication) should be routinely collected. The scope of the health information system should be then gradually broadened to collect routine information on NCD prevalence, intervention, and quality of care from tertiary to primary health facilities.

Policy Options and Strategies for Individual Clinical Interventions for the Treatment of NCDs in the Health Sector

The MOHFW, in collaboration with the private sector, may consider the following actions:

- *Strengthening health service delivery to provide high-quality and effective NCD control and treatment services in selected public health facilities.* The physician and nonphysician workforce will need the treatment guidelines, knowledge, and skills to diagnose and treat NCDs within the primary care system. Pilots to understand best practices and those appropriate for Bangladesh need to be studied. Adequate supply and access to essential medications are needed, especially for the poor. Collaboration with the private sector, NGOs, medical schools, and specialized centers may enhance provision of such services for wider segments of the population. To prevent heart attack and stroke, a "polypill" containing aspirin, beta-blocker, thiazide diuretic, angiotensin-converting enzyme inhibitor, and statin, which costs less than $1 per person a year, may be considered. Table 5.5 provides a list of suggested services for managing acute and chronic cases of stroke, coronary heart diseases, and diabetes, tailored to the different levels of health care in Bangladesh.

- *Developing strategic purchasing mechanisms to motivate public and private service providers to provide cost-effective and high-quality prevention and treatment services.* For example, payments can be linked to performance in the public sector and by private health insurance programs in relation to reduction of NCD risk factors and prevention. Outsourcing expensive and high-tech clinical interventions to the private sector may be more cost effective than in the public sector.

- *Developing and monitoring indicators related to NCD treatment, including conducting impact evaluation studies.* Process, output, and quality indicators related to clinical treatment of NCDs may be included in the relevant operational plans, such as Essential Service Delivery and Improved Hospital Service Management, as well as collected from those health facilities that provide these services.

Note

1. Conventionally, major NCDs include heart disease, stroke, diabetes, cancer, and chronic respiratory diseases (DGHS 2007).

References

Abegunde, D., C. Mathers, T. Adam, M. Ortegon, and K. Strong. 2007. "The Burden and Costs of Chronic Diseases in Low-income and Middle-income Countries." *The Lancet* 370: 1929–38.

BBS (Bangladesh Bureau of Statistics). 2011a. *Report on Sample Vital Registration System 2010.* Dhaka.

———. 2011b. *Preliminary Report on Household Income and Expenditure Survey 2010.* Dhaka.

———. 2012. *Population and Housing Census 2011: Bangladesh at a Glance.* http://www.bbs.gov.bd/WebTestApplication/userfiles/Image/Census2011/Bangladesh_glance.pdf.

BHW (Bangladesh Health Watch). 2008. *The State of Health in Bangladesh 2007: Health Workforce in Bangladesh.* Dhaka: BRAC University.

Choudhury, S., F. Tabassum, J. Ahmed, M. Zaman, A. Rouf, R. Khandaker, and A. Malik. 2010. "Daily Salt Intake Estimated from Urinary Excretion of Sodium in a Bangladeshi Population." Paper presented at World Congress of Cardiology, Beijing, June 16–19.

DGHS (Directorate General of Health Services), MOHFW (Ministry of Health and Family Welfare). 2007. *Strategic Plan for Surveillance and Prevention of Non-Communicable Diseases in Bangladesh 2007–2010*. Dhaka: DGHS, MOHFW.

————. 2008. *National Cancer Control Strategy and Plan of Action 2009–2015*. Dhaka: MOHFW.

Engelgau, M. M., S. El-Saharty, P. Kudesia, V. Rajan, S. Rosenhouse, and K. Okamoto. 2011. *Capitalizing on the Demographic Transition: Tackling Noncommunicable Diseases in South Asia*. Washington, DC: World Bank.

El-Saharty, S., K. Z. Ahsan, A. Ritter, and J. F. May. Forthcoming. "Population, Family Planning and Reproductive Health in Bangladesh: Towards Policy Harmonization." HNP Discussion Paper, World Bank, Washington, DC.

Gottret, P., and G. Schieber. 2010. "Health Financing in South Asia. Health System Objective & Socioeconomic Overview: Achievements & Challenges." Paper presented at the South Asia Regional Forum on Health Financing, Maldives, June 2–4.

Goyal, A., and S. Yusuf. 2006. "The Burden of Cardiovascular Disease in the Indian Subcontinent." *Indian Journal of Medical Research* 124 (September): 235–44.

IHME (Institute for Health Metrics and Evaluation). Forthcoming. *Global Burden of Disease Study 2010. Bangladesh Results by Cause 1990–2010*. Seattle, WA.

Islam, N. 2005. *Dhaka Now*. Dhaka: Bangladesh Geographical Society.

NIPORT (National Institute of Population Research and Training), MEASURE Evaluation, ICDDR,B, and ACPR (National Institute of Population Research and Training, MEASURE Evaluation, International Centre for Diarrhoeal Disease Research, Bangladesh, and Associates for Community and Population Research). 2008. *2006 Bangladesh Urban Health Survey*. Dhaka: NIPORT, ICDDR,B, ACPR; Chapel Hill, NC: MEASURE Evaluation.

NIPORT, Mitra and Associates, and Macro International. 2009. *Bangladesh Demographic and Health Survey 2007*. Dhaka: USAID, NIPORT, Macro International.

NIPORT, Mitra and Associates, and ICF International. 2013. *Bangladesh Demographic and Health Survey 2011*. Dhaka.

Ramaraj, R., and P. Chellappa. 2008. "Cardiovascular Risk in South Asians." *Postgraduate Medical Journal* 84 (996): 518–23.

Streatfield, P. K., and Z. A. Karar. 2008. "Population Challenges for Bangladesh in the Coming Decades." *Journal of Health, Population, and Nutrition* 26 (3): 261–72.

UNICEF (United Nations Children's Fund) and BBS. 2005. *National Low Birth Weight Survey of Bangladesh: 2003–2004*. Dhaka: BBS with assistance from UNICEF.

World Bank. 2013. World DataBank (BETA) World Development Indicators. (accessed January 22, 2013). http://databank.worldbank.org/data/views/reports/tableview.aspx.

WHO (World Health Organization). 2006. *The World Health Report 2006: Working Together for Health. Geneva.* http://www.who.int/whosis/mort/profiles/mort_searo_bgd_bangladesh.pdf.

————. 2008. "Disease and Injury Regional Estimates: Cause-Specific Mortality: Regional Estimates for 2008." http://www.who.int/healthinfo/global_burden_disease/estimates_regional/en/index.html.

————. 2010. "Creating an Enabling Environment for Population-based Salt Reduction Strategies." Geneva, Switzerland: WHO; London: Food Standards Agency. http://whqlibdoc.who.int/publications/2010/9789241500777_eng.pdf.

————. 2011. *WHO Report on the Global Tobacco Epidemic, 2011. Warning about the Dangers of Tobacco*. Geneva.

WHO SEARO (World Health Organization, Regional Office for South East Asia). 2007. *"Impact of Tobacco-Related Illnesses in Bangladesh,"* edited by M. M. Zaman, N. Nargis, A. Perucic, and K. Rahman. New Delhi: WHO SEARO. http://www.ban.searo.who.int/LinkFiles/Publication_Tobacco_Free_Initiative_Health_Cost_ban.pdf.

CHAPTER 1

Contexts and Transitions

Global, Regional, and Country Contexts

A Densely Populated and Poor Country

Bangladesh is the most densely populated large country in the world (UN DESA 2012) and is Asia's fifth and the world's eighth most populous large country (World Bank 2013). With an estimated population of about 150 million in 2011 (World Bank 2013), it is expected to increase to 218 million by 2030 (UN DESA 2008). Yet it is also one of the poorest nations in the world with a per capita gross national income (GNI) of $780 in 2011 (World Bank 2013). In 2010, an estimated 32 percent of the population lived below the national poverty line, albeit an improvement from 57 percent in 1992 (World Bank 2013).

Regional Indicators Vary Widely in South Asia, though Populations Are Largely Rural

From a regional perspective, several country-level contextual factors need consideration for understanding the burden of disease (BOD) and for developing effective responses. Table 1.1 profiles the basic population and health indicators in South Asian countries, and shows wide variations in population size from the small countries of Bhutan and Maldives with less than 1.0 million to India with 1.2 billion. Yet in all countries, the majority of the population lives in rural areas—an important point for the challenges not only of addressing social determinants and risk factors for noncommunicable diseases (NCDs) but also of delivering care.

The range in life expectancy is wide—from 48 years in Afghanistan to 77 years in Maldives. Bangladesh is in the upper mid-range (69 years). Physician and hospital bed density are low in Bangladesh and across the region, with exceptions in Maldives, Nepal, and Sri Lanka (for hospital beds) and Maldives (for physician density), although these two density indicators reflect national averages and do not unmask the heterogeneity in the country, especially between urban and rural areas (see box 1.1).

Total health expenditure ranges from 2.2 percent of gross domestic product (GDP) in Pakistan to 7.6 percent in Afghanistan, with Bangladesh in the lower mid-range (3.5 percent). Spending on health per person in Bangladesh was

---

Box 1.1 Chapter One Summary

- Although still one of the lowest-income countries in the world, Bangladesh has made huge strides in reducing fertility as well as maternal and child mortality, and in increasing life expectancy.
- New population and health challenges stem from rapid demographic and epidemiological transitions, urbanization, the emerging burden of noncommunicable diseases (NCDs), and vulnerability to climate change.

---

around $23 in 2010—inadequate to secure basic services. Private spending, most of which is out of pocket, was high (66 percent of total health expenditure). Such high out-of-pocket spending for services and medications highlights the need to address financing and equity issues (Engelgau *et al.* 2011).

Solid Economic Growth and Generally Positive Social and Health Trends

Despite periods of political turmoil and frequent natural disasters in Bangladesh, the last decade has been marked by sustained growth, stable macroeconomic management, significant poverty reduction, and rapid social transformation and human development. Since the turn of the century, aggregate GDP has been rising at a respectable 5.3 percent a year in real terms, or by 4.0 percent per capita, contributing to a decline in poverty from 49.0 percent in 2000 to 32.0 percent in 2010 (World Bank 2013), in a period when Bangladesh had disproportionate poverty reduction for its growth. The major economic growth factors were expansion in readymade garment exports and remittances from migrant laborers working primarily in unskilled positions in Malaysia and the Middle East.

Strong policy interventions have led to a continuous reduction in annual population growth from 2.3 percent in 1981 to 1.2 percent in 2011 (BBS 2012; World Bank 2013). Bangladesh is a model country in reducing fertility—total fertility was 6.6 children per woman of child-bearing age in the mid-1970s and dropped to 2.3 in 2011 (NIPORT *et al.* 2012). Reversal of past trends of male bias in survival is evident with women now living longer than men (69 versus 67 years in 2010) (BBS 2011).

Between 1990 and 2011, life expectancy rose by 13 years, from 56 to 69 years (BBS 2011; World Bank 2013). Bangladeshis now have a life expectancy of three or four years longer than Indians, despite Indians, on average, having twice their per capita income. Even more encouraging, the improvement in life expectancy has been as great among the poor as the rich.

Literacy and education are further indicators of national health, as well as income-earning potential. In 2008, 48.6 percent of men and 49.1 percent of women over the age of 15 were literate, leading to gender parity, though disparity between urban and rural literacy exists: the rural combined rate is

Table 1.1 Demographic, Economic, and Health Profiles for South Asian Countries, 2011

Category	Indicators	Afghanistan	Bangladesh	Bhutan	India	Maldives	Nepal	Pakistan	Sri Lanka
Population	Total (million)	35.3	**150.5**	0.7	1,241.5	0.3	30.5	176.7	20.7
	Growth (annual %)	2.7	**1.2**	1.7	1.4	1.3	1.7	1.8	1.0
	Rural (% of total)	76.5	**71.6**	64.4	68.7	58.9	83.0	63.8	84.9
	Over 65 years (% of total)	2.3	**4.6**	4.8	5.0	5.2	4.2	4.3	8.4
	Dependency ratio (% of working-age population)								
	Old	4.4	**7.1**	7.3	7.7	7.6	7.0	7.1	12.6
	Young	89.2	**47.4**	43.5	46.6	37.4	58.9	57.3	37.3
Economy	GNI per capita Atlas method (current US$)	470	**780**	2,130	1,410	5,720	540	1,120	2,580
	GNI per capita ($ PPP)	1,140	**1,940**	5,570	3,590	7,430	1,260	2,870	5,520
	Annual growth GDP (%)	5.7	**6.7**	5.6	6.9	7.5	3.9	3.0	8.3
	Labor force participation rate (2010)								
	Female 15 years and older (%)	15.9	**59.8**	68.2	30.3	57.2	83.1	23.0	38.0
	Male 15 years and older (%)	81.9	**86.8**	77.9	83.1	78.4	88.8	85.9	81.1
	Extreme poverty (% <$1.25 PPP)	NA	**43.3[a]**	10.2[f]	32.7[a]	NA	24.8[a]	21.0[e]	7.0[f]
	Poverty headcount ratio at national poverty line (% of population)	36.0[e]	**31.5**	23.2[f]	29.8[a]	NA	25.2	22.3[d]	15.2[f]
Health indicators	Mortality rate, infant (per 1,000 live births)	72.7	**36.7**	42.0	47.4	9.2	39.0	59.2	10.5
	Maternal mortality ratio (national estimate, per 100,000 live births)	1,600[h]	**190[a]**	260[j]	250[d]	140[j]	280[b]	250[f]	39[d]
	Crude death rate (per 1,000 population)	15.9[a]	**6.0**	6.9	8.0	3.6	5.8	7.5[a]	6.6[a]
	Life expectancy (years)	48.3[a]	**68.9**	67.3	65.5	76.9	68.7	65.2[a]	74.7[a]

table continues next page

Table 1.1 Demographic, Economic, and Health Profiles for South Asian Countries, 2011 *(continued)*

Category	Indicators	Afghanistan	Bangladesh	Bhutan	India	Maldives	Nepal	Pakistan	Sri Lanka
Health services	Hospital beds (per 10,000 population)	4[a]	**3**[b]	18	9[b]	43[c]	50[d]	6[a]	31[g]
	Physicians (per 10,000 population, 2010)	2	**3**	0.02	6	16	NA	8	5
Health spending (2010)	Total health expenditure (% of GDP)	7.6	**3.5**	5.2	4.1	6.3	5.5	2.2	2.9
	Per capita total health expenditure ($)	37.7	**23.3**	108.5	54.2	382.5	29.8	21.8	70.0
	Public health expenditure (% of govt. expenditure)	1.6	**7.4**	10.5	3.6	8.6	7.9	3.6	5.8
	Public health expenditure (% of total health expenditure)	11.7	**33.6**	86.8	29.2	60.5	33.2	38.5	44.7

Source: World Bank 2013.

Note: GDP = gross domestic product; GNI = gross national income; PPP = purchasing power parity; NA = Not available.

a. 2010.
b. 2005.
c. 2009.
d. 2006.
e. 2008.
f. 2007.
g. 2004.
h. 2002.
i. 2000.
j. 2001.

46.0 percent compared with 57.0 percent in urban areas (BBS and UNESCO 2008). A larger percentage of females of ages 15–19 have completed primary education (78 percent) than males (69 percent) of the same age group. More than 90 percent of girls enrolled in primary school in 2005, slightly more than boys. That was twice the female enrollment rate in 2000. However, both genders saw decreases between 2004 and 2007 in completion of secondary education: females from 16.4 to 16.0 percent and males from 23.8 to 20.4 percent (NIPORT *et al.* 2009).

During the last few decades, Bangladesh made remarkable progress on most health outcomes, and the country is on track to achieve Millennium Development Goals (MDGs) 4 and 5. The maternal mortality ratio (MMR) declined by 41 percent from 322 maternal deaths per 100,000 live births in 2001 to 190 in 2010 (World Bank 2013). Under-five child mortality rates declined by 29 percent from 51 per 1,000 live births in 2004 to 37 in 2010 (World Bank 2013). These improvements are not a simple result of increases in people's income: Bangladesh remains a poor country, with a per capita GNI of $1,940 in 2011 at purchasing power parity (World Bank 2013). Specific challenges facing the nation include a population characterized by still-high fertility and avoidable mortality, persistent poverty, a geographic location prone to natural disasters, and a state with inefficiencies in governance (Bangladesh News 2008; Paul 2009).

Exacerbating Impact of Urbanization

In 2011, around 28 percent of the population lived in urban areas (World Bank 2013), but according to the 2006 Bangladesh Urban Health Survey, rural-to-urban migration is common, with 6 out of 10 slum migrants and 5 out of 10 non-slum migrants living in a village until age 12 (NIPORT *et al.* 2008). This rapid urbanization is likely to have a major impact on the health profile of the population, as many of these migrants lack human and financial capital in their transition to the city (NIPORT *et al.* 2008).

Bangladesh had one of the highest urban population growth rates (more than 7 percent a year in the urban slums) in the three decades to the late 1990s (Anam, Kabir, and Rai 1993; CUS, NIPORT, and MEASURE Evaluation 2006).

Dhaka, the capital city, is expected to reach a population of 22 million by 2025, making it the third-largest megacity in the South Asia region and among the top 10 largest cities in the world (NIPORT *et al.* 2008). In the mid-2000s, an estimated 37 percent of Dhaka's population (of over 9 million people) lived in slums (Islam 2005). Dhaka continues to grow, at around 320,000 people a year, with more than three-quarters migrating to urban slums or areas with even less shelter (Streatfield and Karar 2008). Employment, shelter, and basic services accessible to the growing number of urban poor is an emerging socioeconomic issue yet to be fully addressed by policy makers (Koehlmoos *et al.* 2009).

In almost every major urban center of Bangladesh, tens of thousands of people live in overcrowded slums, streets, or other public places that lack basic facilities such as safe water, sanitation, and health services (Koehlmoos *et al.* 2009; Streatfield and Karar 2008). Urban slums are more likely to flood during the rainy season (30 percent) than urban non-slums (18 percent) or district munici- palities (22 percent). Across the three urban domains, a majority of non-slum households (80 percent) had a system to dispose of sewage properly, followed by district municipalities (41 percent) and slums (30 percent). Availability of a health program or a services center was highest in district municipalities (86 percent), then non-slums (64 percent) and slums (51 percent) (NIPORT *et al.* 2008).

Demographic and Epidemiological Transitions

Aging Population Is on the Rise

Key for a nation making decisions in light of a potential increase in the burden of NCDs is that the projected elderly population (the share aged 60 years or more) will increase hugely, such that the elderly will make up 18.8 percent of the total population by mid-century (figure 1.1).

Bangladesh is projected to undergo a huge demographic transition over the next 50 years with a substantial decline among the proportion of the population under 15 years and of females of reproductive age. This transition stems from

Figure 1.1 Population in the 21st Century, Bangladesh
Million

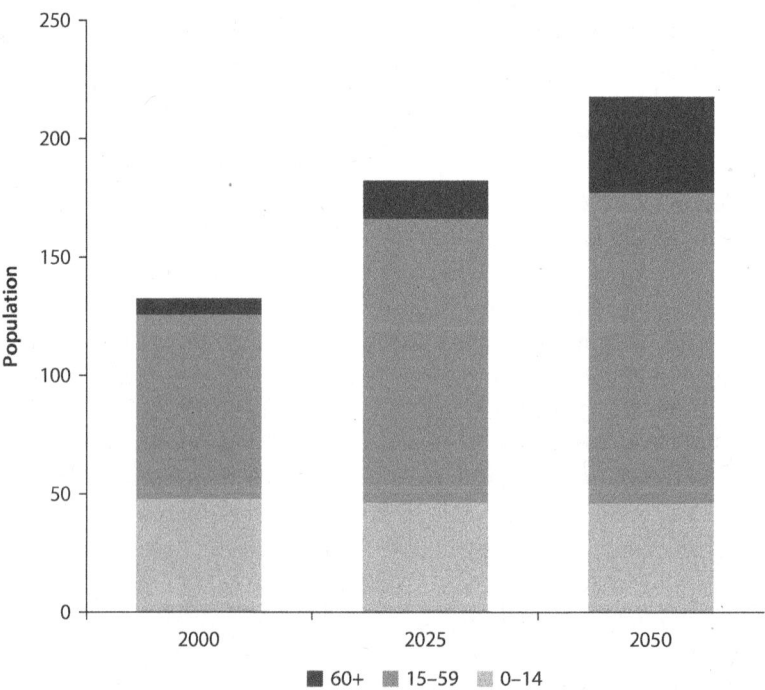

Source: Modified from Streatfield and Karar 2008.

the trend of reduction in the total fertility rate (TFR) and trends in other population indicators (El-Saharty *et al.* forthcoming). The constrictive population structure projected for Bangladesh in 2051 is evident in figure 1.2.

These demographic changes will have a serious impact on health expenditure (figure 1.3) for the countries across South Asia. For Bangladesh, the increase in health spending between 2000 and 2020 due to population growth will be 29.7 percent and due to aging about 18.0 percent, for an overall rise of

Figure 1.2 Changing Age Structure of the Population in Bangladesh, 2001, 2026, and 2051

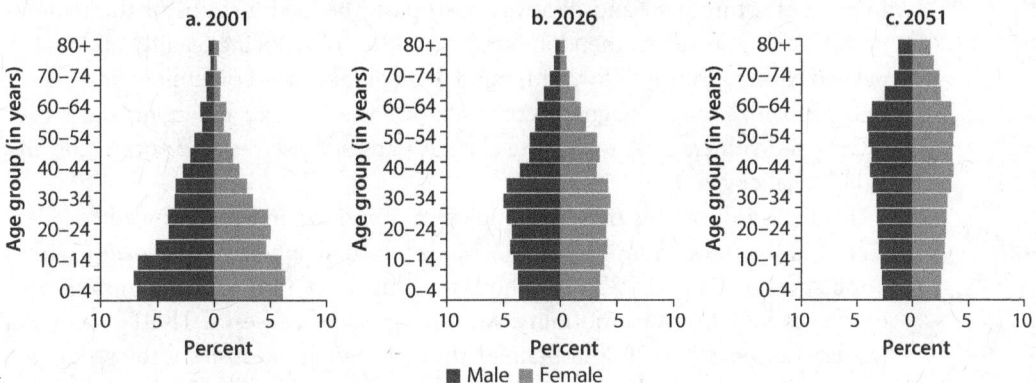

Source: El-Saharty *et al.* forthcoming.

Figure 1.3 Projected Impact of Population Growth and Aging on Total Health Expenditure in the South Asia Region, 2000–20

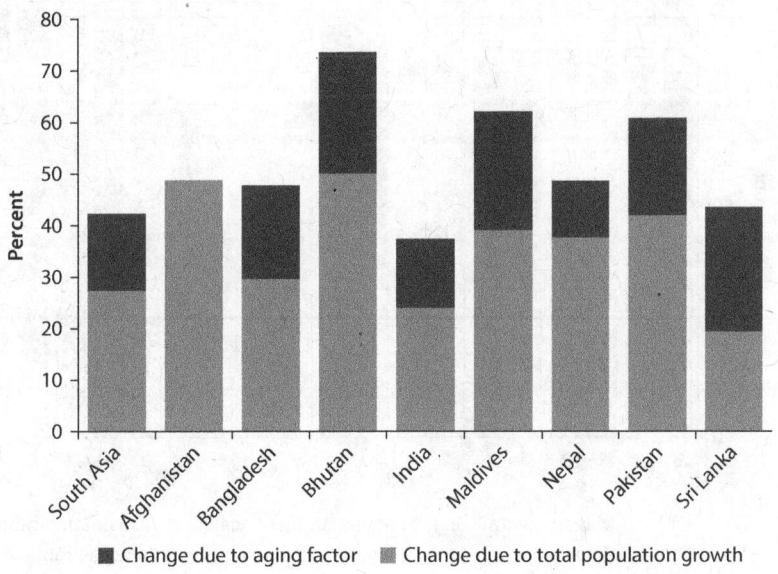

Source: Gottret and Schieber 2010.

about 47.7 percent. This health spending increase will be exacerbated by the trends in NCDs (chapter 2). The demographic transition will also result in a huge middle-age bulge in the population structure, which will have a large impact on the NCD burden—studies[1] have already established that a substantial proportion of NCDs arise during middle age rather than in the elderly age group. A rapid rise in the middle- and working-age population, and existing trends of migration to urban areas, will have a compounding effect on the NCD burden in the coming years.

Emerging Challenges from the Epidemiological Transition

In spite of a turbulent and disadvantaged past, the health status of the nation's population has made tremendous strides in terms of reducing fertility and maternal and child mortality. Now, with rapid demographic and epidemiological transitions, urbanization, a stagnant contraceptive use rate, an emerging burden of NCDs, and vulnerability to climate change, Bangladesh faces new population and health challenges.

Figure 1.4 illustrates the epidemiological transition in rural Bangladesh. Data collected for more than 40 years in Matlab, a rural subdistrict (*upazila*) with a population of around 222,000, show the shift over time from communicable disease to NCD-related mortality. An assessment of causes of 18,917 deaths in Matlab during 1986–2006, obtained through verbal autopsies, shows that the proportion of deaths due to communicable diseases fell from 52 to 11 percent, while that due to NCDs rose from 8 to 68 percent.

Figure 1.4 NCD Mortality Increases in Rural Bangladesh (Matlab), 1986–2006

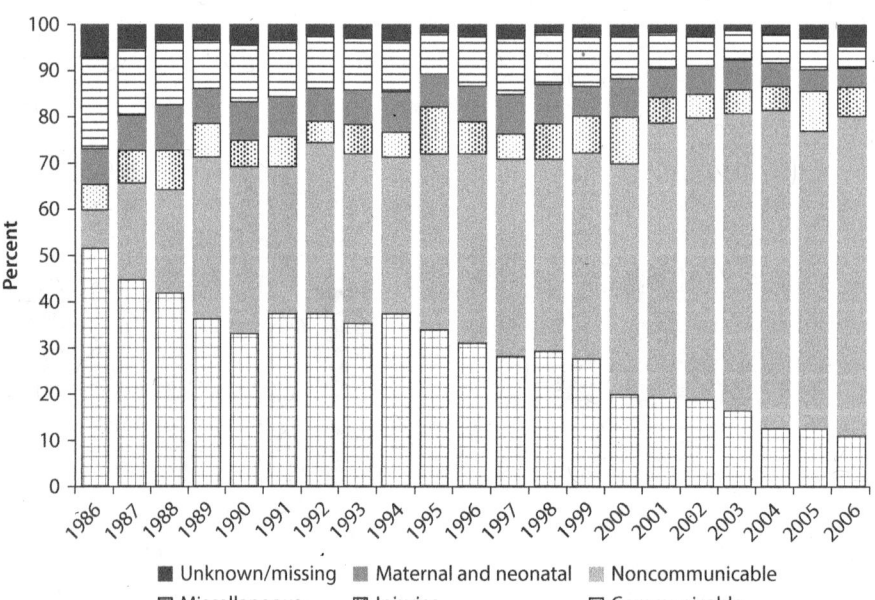

Source: Karar, Alam, and Streatfield 2009.

Note

1. http://www.chp.gov.hk/files/pdf/grp-hkphps-vii_non-communicable%20diseases_en.pdf.

References

Anam, S., R. Kabir, and P. Rai. 1993. *Staying Alive: Urban Poor in Bangladesh*, edited by R. Kabir and P. Rai. Dhaka: United Nations Children's Fund.

Bangladesh News. 2008. "Kissinger Declines Comment on 'Basket Case.'" Dhaka, January 27.

BBS (Bangladesh Bureau of Statistics). 2011. *Report on Sample Vital Registration System 2010*. Dhaka.

———. 2012. *Population and Housing Census 2011: Bangladesh at a Glance*. http://www.bbs.gov.bd/WebTestApplication/userfiles/Image/Census2011/Bangladesh_glance.pdf.

BBS, and UNESCO (Bangladesh Bureau of Statistics and United Nations Educational, Scientific, and Cultural Organization). 2008. *Literacy Assessment Survey 2008*. Dhaka.

CUS, NIPORT, and MEASURE Evaluation (Centre for Urban Studies, National Institute of Population Research and Training, and MEASURE Evaluation). 2006. *Slums of Urban Bangladesh: Mapping and Census, 2005*. Dhaka: NIPORT; Chapel Hill, NC: MEASURE Evaluation.

El-Saharty, S., K. Z. Ahsan, A. Ritter, and J. F. May. Forthcoming. "Population, Family Planning and Reproductive Health in Bangladesh: Towards Policy Harmonization." HNP Discussion Paper, World Bank, Washington, DC.

Engelgau, M. M., S. El-Saharty, P. Kudesia, V. Rajan, S. Rosenhouse, and K. Okamoto. 2011. *Capitalizing on the Demographic Transition: Tackling Noncommunicable Diseases in South Asia*. Washington, DC: World Bank.

Gottret, P., and G. Schieber. 2010. "Health Financing in South Asia. Health System Objective & Socioeconomic Overview: Achievements & Challenges." Paper presented at the South Asia Regional Forum on Health Financing, Maldives, June 2–4.

Islam, N. 2005. *Dhaka Now*. Dhaka: Bangladesh Geographical Society.

Karar, Z. A., N. Alam, and P. K. Streatfield. 2009. "Epidemiologic Transition in Rural Bangladesh, 1968–2006." *Global Health Action* 2.

Koehlmoos, T., M. J. Uddin, A. Ashraf, and M. Rashid. 2009. "Homeless in Dhaka: Violence, Sexual Harassment, and Drug-Abuse." *Journal of Health, Population and Nutrition* 27 (4): 452–61.

NIPORT, MEASURE Evaluation, ICDDR,B and ACPR (National Institute of Population Research and Training, MEASURE Evaluation, International Centre for Diarrhoeal Disease Research, Bangladesh, and Associates for Community and Population Research). 2008. *2006 Bangladesh Urban Health Survey*. Dhaka: NIPORT, ICDDR,B, ACPR; Chapel Hill, NC: MEASURE Evaluation.

NIPORT, Mitra and Associates, and Macro International. 2009. *Bangladesh Demographic and Health Survey 2007*. Dhaka: USAID, NIPORT, Macro International.

NIPORT, Mitra and Associates, and MEASURE DHS ICF. 2012. *Bangladesh Demographic and Health Survey 2011: Preliminary Report*. Dhaka.

Paul, S. 2009. "Potential Bangladesh and Road to One-Party Rule." *Modern Ghana*, Accra, April 4. http://www.modernghana.com/news/209806/1/potential-bangladesh-and-road-to-one-party-rule.html.

Streatfield, P. K., and Z. A. Karar. 2008. "Population Challenges for Bangladesh in the Coming Decades." *Journal of Health, Population, and Nutrition* 26 (3): 261–72.

UN DESA (United Nations Department of Economic and Social Affairs Population Division). 2008. *World Urbanization Prospects: The 2007 Revision.* New York: United Nations.

———. 2012. *2011 Demographic Yearbook.* New York: United Nations.

World Bank. 2013. World DataBank (BETA) World Development Indicators (accessed January 22, 2013). http://databank.worldbank.org/data/views/reports/tableview.aspx.

CHAPTER 2

Burden of Disease and Risk Factors for NCDs

Global and Regional Burden of NCDs

NCDs Are Now a Greater Burden Than Communicable Diseases

Globally, the burden of disease (BOD) has been shifting toward noncommunicable diseases (NCDs) over the last two decades (see box 2.1). The Global Burden of Disease Study 2010 documented that during 1990–2010, among the top five causes of forgone disability-adjusted life years (DALYs), only the NCDs like ischemic heart disease and stroke increased in terms of their global burden, and ischemic heart disease has become the leading cause (figure 2.1). Among the top five risk factors for poor health globally, high blood pressure and tobacco use have become the top two.

In South Asia, the BOD is shifting fast as well. In 2010, NCDs and injuries accounted for 57.0 percent, up from 37.9 percent in 1990, and a larger proportion than communicable diseases, maternal and child health illnesses, and nutrition causes combined, which accounted for 43.0 percent (figure 2.2).

This pattern is similar to that of high-income countries decades ago. These countries are now well advanced into their demographic and epidemiological transitions, with most of their BOD due to NCDs, which account for 95 percent of DALYs (box 2.2).

The country-level BOD for NCDs in South Asia is quite variable: total DALYs lost due to NCDs are estimated to range from 87 percent in Sri Lanka (similar to the pattern found in middle- and high-income countries) to 46 percent in Afghanistan (figure 2.3).

A study of 52 countries, including Bangladesh, India, Nepal, Pakistan, and Sri Lanka, found that the populations of the South Asia region were six years younger (53 versus 59 years) than those in the rest of the world at the time of their first heart attack, had high levels of risk factors such as diabetes and high cholesterol, and had low levels of protective factors (physical activity and dietary habits). Thus, this greater susceptibility to NCDs in South Asia suggests that NCDs may have a greater impact than in other regions (Goyal and Yusuf 2006; Ramaraj and Chellappa 2008).

Box 2.1 Chapter Two Summary

- The BOD pattern is now similar to that of high-income countries decades ago.
- The major causes of mortality from NCDs are cardiovascular diseases (CVDs), cancer, respiratory diseases, injuries, and diabetes.
- All these NCDs but injuries are linked to a few common risk factors, namely high tobacco use, air pollution (including indoor fires for cooking and heating), poor diet and nutrition, occupational risks, high blood pressure, malnutrition and low birth weight, lack of physical activity, and alcohol consumption and substance abuse.
- Highlights of the NCD burden and associated risk factors are: 7.3 percent of the population has CVDs; 66 percent of cancer patients are of working age; the country has some of the highest tobacco use in the world among both men and women; salt intake is high; the rate of low birth weight (36 percent) is among the highest in the world; and more than 40 percent of children under five are either underweight or moderately stunted.
- Over 20 years, Bangladesh has made huge gains in the basic condition of people's lives, helped by disproportionate poverty reduction relative to GDP growth. However, NCDs can hold back economic development and efforts to reduce poverty.
- As the burden of NCDs varies across socioeconomic strata and gender, policy makers should consider the economic and social impacts of the NCD epidemic in formulating NCD-related policies, particularly for the poor.

Figure 2.1 Main Causes of Global DALYs and Top Five Risk Factors for Poor Health, 1990 and 2010

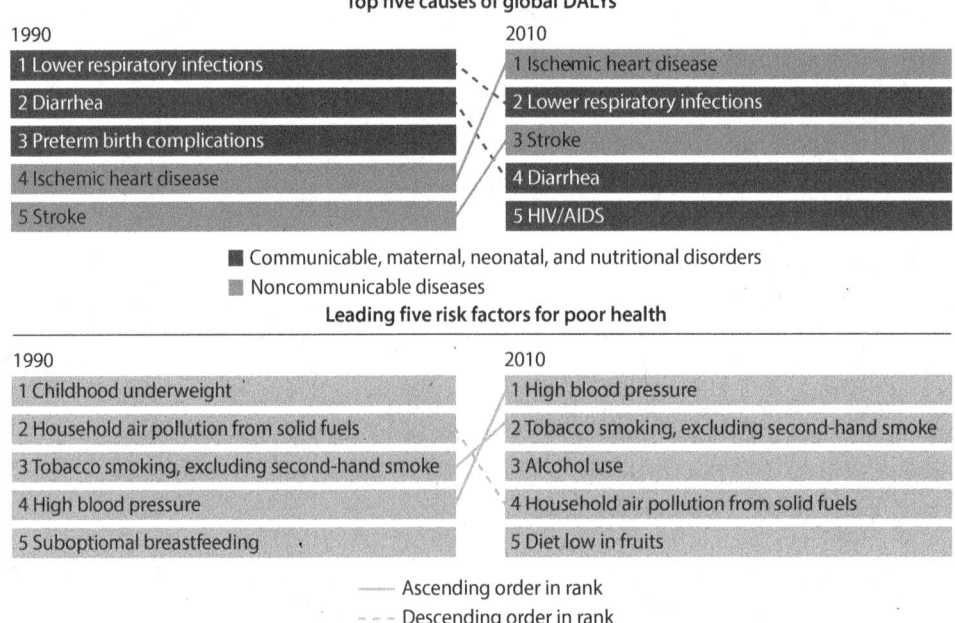

Source: Watts and Cairncross 2012.
Note: DALY = disability-adjusted life years; HIV/AIDS = human immunodeficiency virus/acquired immune deficiency syndrome.

Figure 2.2 BOD as a Proportion of Total Forgone DALYs by Cause, Global and South Asia, 2010

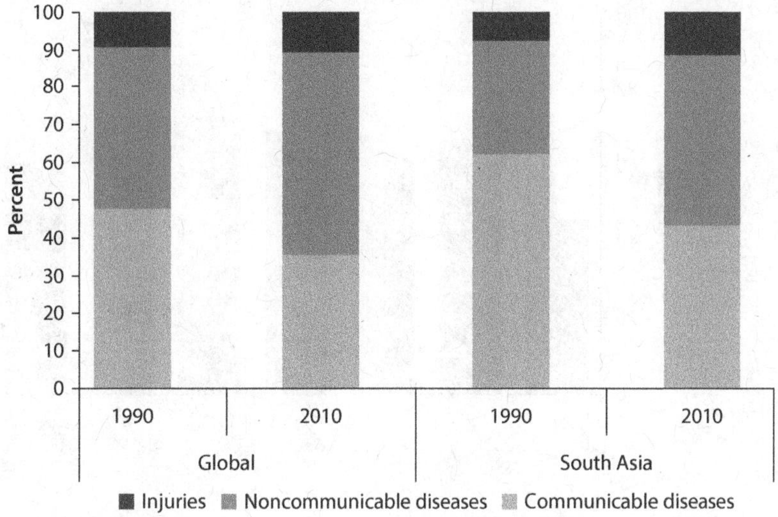

Source: Murray et al. 2012.
Note: BOD = burden of disease; DALY = disability-adjusted life years.

Box 2.2 Methods to Describe the Health Situation in South Asia

Mortality data in the region are scant. Therefore, to describe the health situation, we use undiscounted DALYs, which measure the number of years a person would lose due to disability and premature mortality. Death rates are presented where possible.

A number of health surveys have been carried out in the region; they are very useful at the country level, but often not comparable at the regional level. An advantage of using DALYs to measure the BOD is that it considers years with disability and thus it includes conditions that, although not fatal, can be a large economic and social burden. Other benefits of DALYs are that they have been used around the world and that there is a global commitment to continue providing and adjusting these estimates.

Yet South Asian researchers have raised concern over the weights used to measure disability, since they have not been fully validated in the region. In addition, for countries with no data, DALYs have been calculated by extrapolating the level and composition of death and disability from countries of similar epidemiologic and economic profiles, allowing us to assess only by broad groups of diseases and leading conditions within those groups. And, because of the methodology used to estimate DALYs, the death of a child contributes more DALYs than the death of an older person.

But despite these caveats, DALY estimates have been reasonably close when compared with new data, such as those from surveys or special studies. However, more work is needed on collecting and analyzing NCD data in South Asia.

Tackling Noncommunicable Diseases in Bangladesh • http://dx.doi.org/10.1596/978-0-8213-9920-0

Figure 2.3 Proportion of Total Deaths and Forgone DALYs Due to NCDs, South Asia, 2004

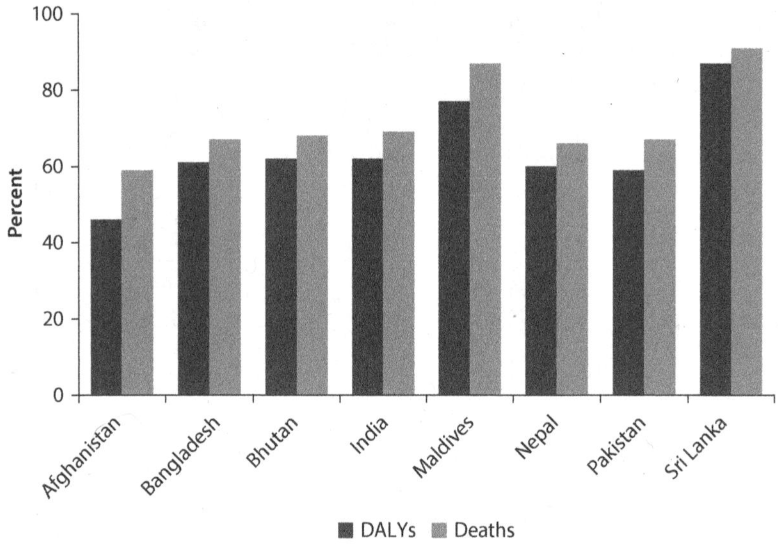

Source: WHO 2008a.
Note: DALYs are age standardized to facilitate country comparisons. DALY = disability-adjusted life years;
NCD = noncommunicable disease.

Bangladesh NCD Burden

Facing the Double Burden

Bangladesh—like many countries in transition—is straddling the demographic and epidemiological transitions.[1] Among 23 developing countries studied, Bangladesh ranked ninth in rates of age-standardized mortality due to chronic diseases, primarily cardiovascular diseases (CVDs) and diabetes (Abegunde *et al.* 2007). Some 68 percent of deaths in Bangladesh are due to NCDs and other chronic health conditions including old age complications (BBS 2011a); a study conducted in medical college hospitals in the country found that about one-third of hospital admissions among patients aged 30 years and over were due to major NCDs[2] (DGHS 2007).

As the burden shifts from surviving birth, childhood, and childbirth, so must the focus of the country's health system shift to continue to meet the needs of the population, particularly the poor. An annual "reality check" study of the ultra-poor by the Swedish International Development Cooperation Agency reports that demand is increasing for care for diabetes, heart disease, and stress in Bangladesh (SIDA 2009). However, there is no free or subsidized treatment for NCDs through the government health system, unlike for some communicable diseases and maternal and child health programs. Even though all health services are, in principle, free in the public sector, the lack of drugs and indirect costs (such as transportation) result in high out-of-pocket spending by NCD patients.

An interesting comparison can be made between risk factors and DALYs. Chronic diseases, except injuries, are estimated to be responsible for almost half of all deaths and 24.1 percent of the BOD measured in DALYs. Although the leading causes of mortality in Bangladesh are predominantly associated with chronic diseases, the risk factors accounting for the greatest number of lost DALYs are mostly associated with communicable diseases, limited access to safe drinking water, and malnutrition, which tend to take young lives (figure 2.3). This figure highlights the challenges that face Bangladesh in tackling NCDs: it must continue to improve its traditional public health functions centered on maternal and child health, while strengthening prevention and management of the conditions that cause the greatest mortality, primarily among adult men and women.

The leading causes of mortality and morbidity, and risk factors in Bangladesh (2010 estimates) are shown in figures 2.4 and 2.5. The figures indicate that Bangladesh is characterized by the "double burden" of communicable and NCDs—a phenomenon in the majority of developing countries (Boutayeb and Boutayeb 2005). People in such countries not only face higher risk of premature death but also of living a longer part of their life in poor health (WHO 2003).

Cardiovascular Diseases—The Biggest Killer

Due to the lack of a good surveillance system, there are few population-based data on CVD. The national Sample Vital Registration System (SVRS) of the national statistical agency, the Bangladesh Bureau of Statistics (BBS), estimates

Figure 2.4 Leading Causes of Mortality and Morbidity in Bangladesh, 2010 Estimates

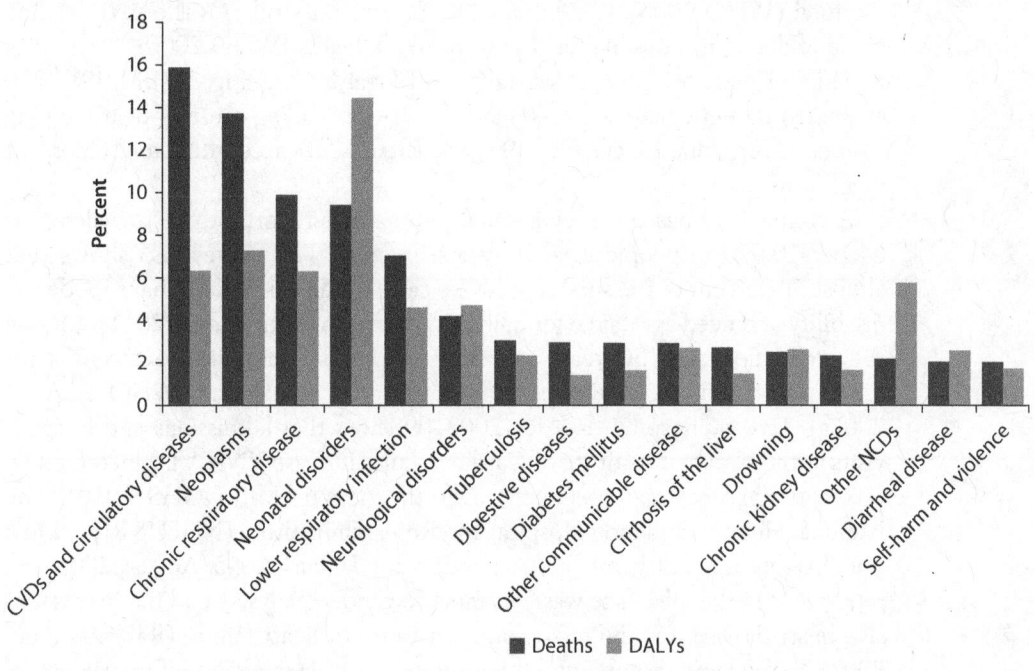

Source: IHME forthcoming.
Note: See appendix 1 for a detailed table. CVD = cardiovascular disease; DALYs = disability-adjusted life years; NCD = noncommunicable disease; CVD = cardiovascular disease.

Figure 2.5 Leading Causes of Premature Deaths in Bangladesh, 2010 Estimates

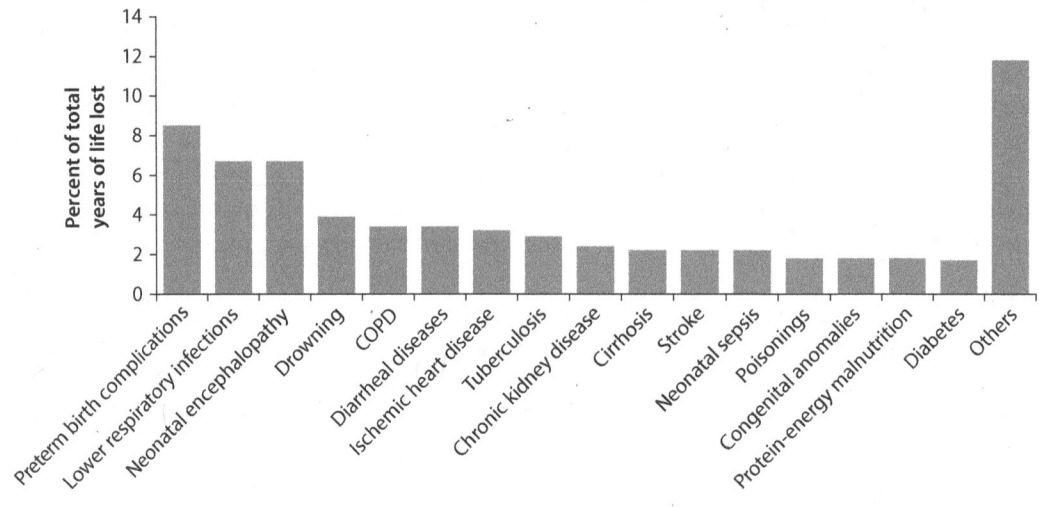

Source: IHME forthcoming.
Note: COPD = chronic obstructive pulmonary disease.

that cardio- and cerebrovascular diseases combined are the major causes of death, followed by asthma and respiratory diseases (BBS 2011a). CVD has an age-standardized mortality rate of 411 per 100,000 (WHO 2009a). Ischemic heart disease is the leading cause of death in Bangladesh, responsible for 12 percent of the total (WHO 2006). Cerebrovascular disease (or stroke) is the sixth leading cause of death, responsible for 6 percent of all deaths (WHO 2006).

The Bangladesh Maternal Mortality and Health Care Survey (BMMS) 2010 estimated that circulatory diseases are the second leading cause of death among women of reproductive age (15–49 years) (figure 2.6), accounting for 16 percent of all deaths.

A community-based survey in rural populations reports stroke prevalence as 64 per 10,000 in people aged 30 years or more. This survey also shows that almost 50 percent of the surviving stroke cases in the community have moderate disability and need assistance for daily activities (Choudhury *et al.* 2011). Among the population aged 30 years and above, ischemic heart disease accounts for 7.7 percent and stroke 8.9 percent of hospital admissions (WHO SEARO 2007a). Tertiary hospital data for 2003–09 show that admissions and outdoor visits at the National Institute of Cardiovascular Diseases (NICVD) increased by 107 and 75 percent, respectively, over the period (MIS-DGHS 2010). The National Heart Foundation Hospital and Research Institute (NHFH&RI) studied the characteristics of heart failure patients for January 2005–August 2006 and reported that the mean age was 54 years (no gender analysis), and that hypertensive heart disease was the most common cause of heart failure (Kabiruzzaman 2007). Several community- and school-based surveys showed that prevalence of rheumatic fever and rheumatic heart disease had been declining (Choudhury *et al.* 2006).

Figure 2.6 Causes of Deaths among Women of Reproductive Age (15–49 Years), Bangladesh, 2010

Percent

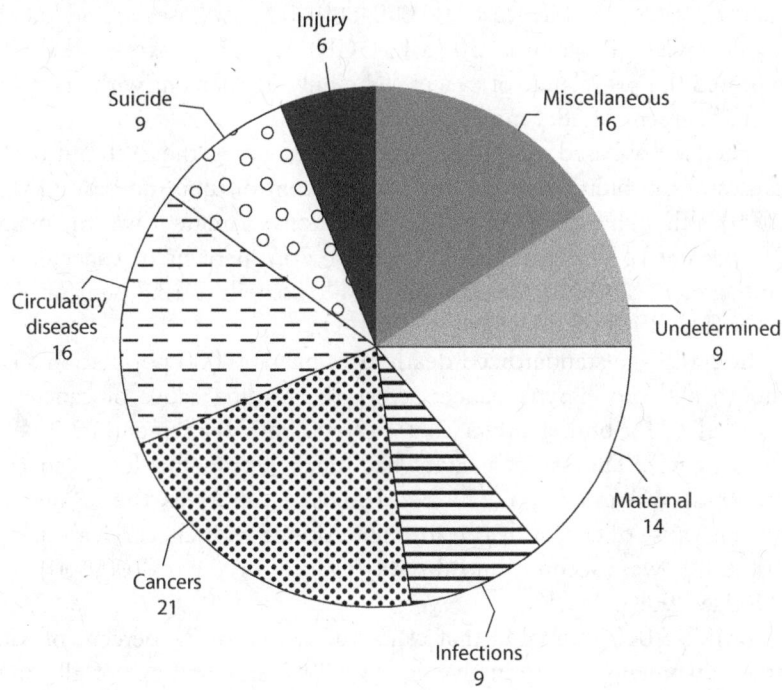

Source: NIPORT *et al.* 2011.

The Bangladesh Household Income and Expenditure Survey (HIES) 2010 collected information on chronic illnesses and duration of ailment from households. According to the preliminary report, 7.3 percent of the population had chronic heart disease, with no real difference in prevalence between urban and rural populations. The average duration of ailment due to chronic heart disease was 75.4 months (BBS 2011b).

A hospital-based cross-sectional study on 14,009 patients at a tertiary cardiac hospital in Dhaka city found that 14.1 percent of patients were diagnosed as heart failure patients and the mean age of hospitalization was 54.1 years—much lower than other related studies conducted outside Bangladesh. More than one-third of the patients (35.8 percent) had ischemic heart disease as the principal etiological factor, but this frequently coexisted with a history of hypertension (46.8 percent). Diabetes coexisted with ischemic heart disease in 41.4 percent of patients (Kabiruzzaman *et al.* 2010).

Cancer—A Heavy Economic Price, Too

According to the National Cancer Control Strategy and Plan of Action 2009–15, cancer is a high priority for Bangladesh because of its economic impact. Most (66 percent) cancer patients are of working age (30–65 years) and can be lost to the nation's workforce prematurely (DGHS 2008). There is no national cancer registry, although information is reported from specialty institutions, public health hospitals, and outpatient facilities. Bangladesh has an estimated 4 million cancer patients, and at least 200,000–800,000 new cases are added every year (Cancer Care Program 2010; MIS-DGHS 2009). However, the HIES 2010 reported the prevalence of cancer to be only 0.4 percent with an average duration of ailment of 58.4 months (BBS 2011b).

The facility-based morbidity profile has cancer as the 29th out of 30 leading causes of morbidity, representing 0.01 percent of total morbidity (MIS-DGHS 2009), although overall population projections estimate it was the main cause in 7.5 percent of deaths in 2005. In 2008, 70.7 percent of cancer deaths were among men; cancer deaths are projected to constitute 12.7 percent of deaths by 2030 (DGHS 2008; Engelgau et al. 2011).

In 2005, age-standardized death rates per 100,000 population suggest that mouth and oropharynx cancers were the leading cause of cancer deaths in Bangladesh for both genders (27.0 per 100,000 for men and 22.5 per 100,000 for women). The same analysis had trachea/bronchus/lung cancer (25 per 100,000) and esophagus (11 per 100,000) cancer as the second and third leading cause of cancer deaths for men. Among women, cervical cancer (21 per 100,000) was second and breast cancer (16 per 100,000) was third (DGHS 2008).

BMMS 2010 estimated that cancer accounts for 21 percent of total deaths among women of reproductive age (13–49 years), and out of all the causes of death among women of reproductive age, only those for cancer increased over the previous decade (figure 2.7).

The flagship public institution for cancer-related services is the National Institute of Cancer Research and Hospital (NICRH) in Dhaka, with an estimated capacity of some 100,000 cancer patients a year. NICRH's most frequently reported cancers are respiratory system (22.2 percent); digestive organ (20.8 percent); breast (12.7 percent); female genital organs (12.1 percent); and lip, oral cavity, and pharynx (10.9 percent) (MIS-DGHS 2009). Together, the burden of female-related cancers is greater than the leading cause of cancer admissions (respiratory system) so that special emphasis is given here to female-related cancers.

Bangladesh reported that less than 5 percent of women aged 50–69 were screened with mammography in the three years prior to the World Health Survey (2000–03). The low rate was typical for low-income countries where no equity analysis (to look at the distribution of mammography screening across the population) was performed (WHO 2008a).

Of the global burden of cervical cancer, one-third of cases are in South Asia, yet no strategies for prevention, screening, or treatment—let alone efforts to target high-risk groups—have been well developed (Sankaranarayanan et al. 2008). A small study (n = 472) of histopathology of cases in the Mymensing district (Dhaka division) found that cervical cancer was the leading cancer among females (Talukdar et al. 2007).

Figure 2.7 Causes of Mortality among Women of Reproductive Age in Bangladesh, 2001 and 2010

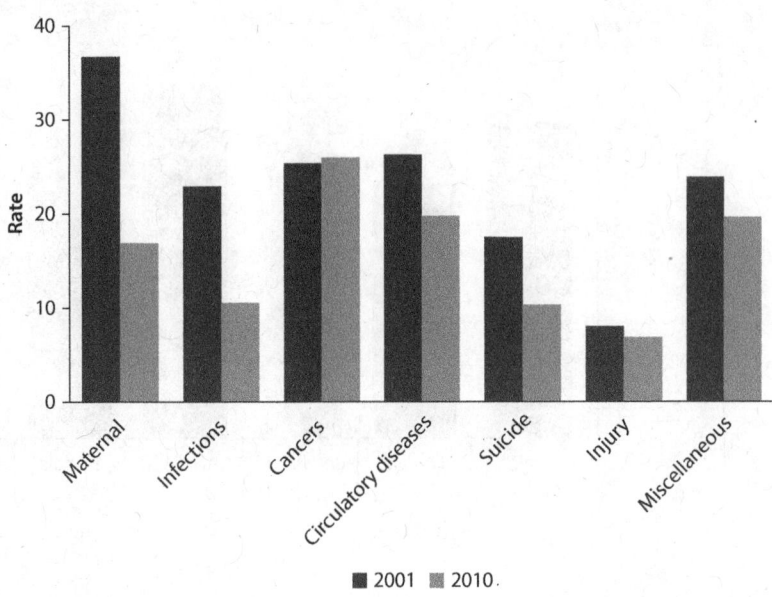

Source: NIPORT et al. 2011.

Respiratory Diseases—Taking a Heavy Toll

In 2004, asthma and other chronic respiratory diseases accounted for 823 DALYs lost per 100,000 population in Bangladesh (WHO 2008a). In 2002, the study of a small national sample estimated a 6.9 percent prevalence of asthma. Other countries in the region have high estimates: using British Medical Research Council (MRC) criteria (CACB 1965) for cough, on most days of the week for three months of the year for at least two years, the reported overall prevalence of chronic obstructive pulmonary disease (COPD) was 18.3 percent among those 20 years or older in Nepal, and 7.7 percent in those 15 years or older in India (Pandey 1984; Qureshi 1994). In Bangladesh, the prevalence of COPD has yet to be estimated at the national level. Small-scale studies indicate that the prevalence among people aged 30 years and above is 3 percent; however, it is 6 percent among patients in medical colleges (WHO SEARO 2007a).

The prevalence data on COPD also vary widely depending on the source and definition of COPD (Celli et al. 2003). Although according to a World Health Organization (WHO) report worldwide prevalence of COPD was estimated at 0.8 percent (Murray and Lopez 1997), well-designed studies have shown prevalence between 4 percent and 10 percent and that is the rate expected in populations where smoking prevalence is high and exposure to biomass fuel is a significant risk factor, as in Bangladesh (Halbert et al. 2003). In 2010, HIES found asthma/respiratory diseases to be among the top five chronic illnesses in Bangladesh. Nationwide, 8.9 percent of the population—10.2 percent of males and 7.7 percent of females—suffered from respiratory diseases during

Figure 2.8 Distribution of People Who Suffered from Asthma/Respiratory Diseases in the Preceding 12 Months by Locality, Bangladesh, 2005 and 2010

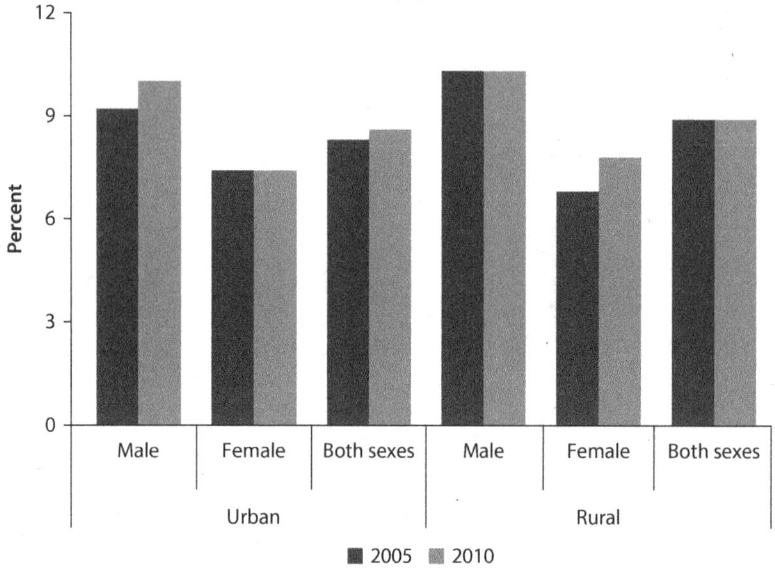

Source: BBS 2011b.

the 12 months preceding the survey (figure 2.8). The average duration of ailment for asthma/respiratory diseases was one of the longest among all the chronic diseases—107.1 months (BBS 2011b).

Injuries—Killing Over 80 Children a Day

In 2010, HIES reported that 3.9 percent of the population in Bangladesh suffered from injury/disability with wide variations by region (4.5 percent rural and 2.2 percent urban) and gender (5 percent males and 3 percent females). The average duration of ailment for injury/disability was 74.5 months (BBS 2011b).

Among children 1–17 years old, injuries are the largest killer, accounting for 38 percent of all classifiable deaths. This means that 83 children a day die of injuries. The leading types of injury-related deaths among children are drowning (59.3 percent), road traffic accidents (12.3 percent), animal bites (9.3 percent), and suicide (8.0 percent). Injuries permanently disable an estimated 13,000 children a year. Around one million children a year suffer nonfatal injuries (ICMH *et al.* 2005). Figure 2.9 shows the five leading causes of death among children due to injuries by type and age group: children 1–4 and 5–9 age groups are most likely to die from drowning at the rate of 86.3 and 26.0 per 100,000 child deaths, respectively. In the 10–14 year age group, road traffic accidents account for 7.5 deaths per 100,000 children, and in the 15–17 age group suicide accounts for 24 deaths per 100,000 children (ICMH *et al.* 2005).

Injuries have an age-standardized mortality rate of 100 per 100,000 (WHO 2009a). In 2002, the overall estimates were that road traffic accidents accounted

Figure 2.9 Death Rate in Each Age Group from the Five Leading Injury Causes among Children

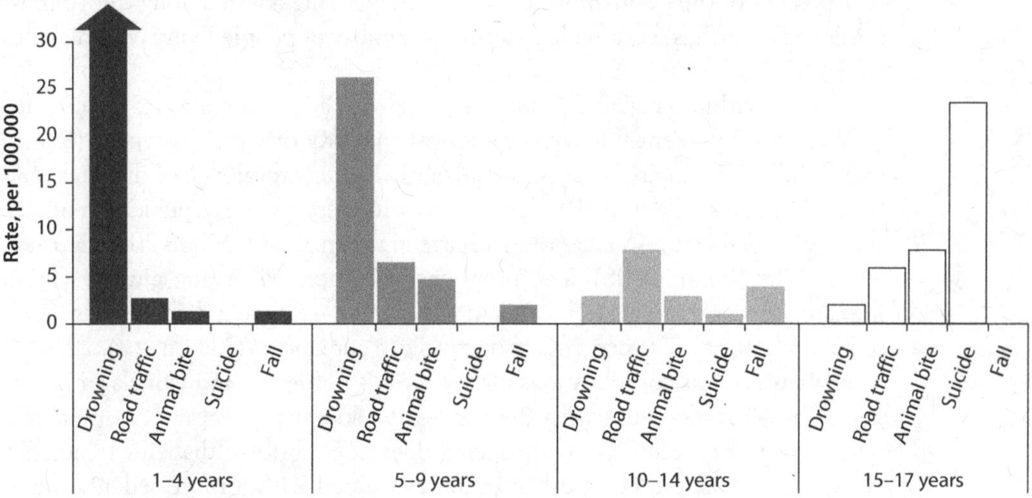

Source: ICMH *et al.* 2005.

for 2 percent of all deaths (19,000). Yet police reports in 2006 only captured 3,160 traffic fatalities (WHO 2009b). Nearly 90 percent of road traffic fatalities were among males and 11 percent among females (WHO 2009b), with a steady increase over time. Road accidents are the most common cause of serious injury for men and are responsible for 40–45 percent of all serious injuries in urban areas among slum and non-slum residents (NIPORT *et al.* 2008). Fifty-four percent of deaths are among pedestrians (WHO 2009b). There is national legislation (the Motor Vehicle Ordinance) on speed limits, drunk driving, motorcycle helmets, and seatbelts, but implementation is very weak. No child-restraint laws in vehicles are in place.

Self-inflicted injuries accounted for 2 percent (17,000) of all deaths in 2002 (WHO 2006). The leading cause of injuries among women is domestic accidents. In the 2006 Bangladesh Urban Health Survey, 57 percent of women reported serious injuries due to domestic accidents, 60 percent in non-slum areas and 64 percent in district municipalities. Forty-two percent of urban slum-dwelling women who had ever experienced domestic violence reported they had suffered an injury as a result of that violence. Non-slum urban women (35.3 percent) and women in district municipalities (30.5 percent) reported slightly lower numbers of injury from domestic violence (NIPORT *et al.* 2008). BMMS 2010 estimated that injuries and suicide account for 6 and 9 percent, respectively, of the total number of deaths among women of reproductive age (13–49 years) (NIPORT *et al.* 2011).

Diabetes—Taking Bangladesh into the 10 Most Burdened Countries

Diabetes is one of the more devastating chronic NCDs, having serious health, economic, and social consequences (IDF 2006a). In 2007, the International Diabetes Federation (IDF) estimated that 3.8 million (4.8 percent of the population) had diabetes, and this number is expected to grow to 7.4 million (6.1 percent of the population) by 2025, placing Bangladesh among the 10 most burdened countries worldwide in terms of number of people living with diabetes (IDF 2006b).

Sources within Bangladesh estimate prevalence at 6.9 percent: 7.5 percent for males and 6.5 percent for females, the vast majority of which is type 2 (Rahim et al. 2007).[3] Urban areas have a significantly higher prevalence of diabetes than rural areas: rates vary from 10.0 percent in some reports to 8.1 percent in others. The risk of diabetes also increases with age in urban areas (DGHS 2007; Hussain et al. 2005; Rahim 2008). The prevalence of impaired fasting glucose (IFG), impaired glucose tolerance (IGT), and newly detected type 2 diabetes was found to be 1.3, 2.0, and 7.0 percent, respectively, in rural areas (Rahim et al. 2010).

Diabetes and its complications place a serious burden on individuals and families in low-income countries where access to adequate treatment is poor and where government and donor financing does not subsidize diabetes treatment. An aging population, rapid urbanization associated with a more sedentary lifestyle, and an altered diet consisting of more energy-dense processed foods (replacing traditional healthy foods) put Bangladesh at risk for increased obesity and the emergence of diabetes. This pattern is also observed in developed economies (WHO 2005).

Studies conducted at a tertiary diabetes hospital in Dhaka estimated that of 473.43 DALYs forgone due to diabetes, only 20.5 percent was due to diabetes itself while the rest (79.5 percent) was due to its complications. The study also estimated that the most number of DALYs forgone were incurred by diabetes with CVDs (37.6 percent), followed by diabetes with retinopathy (19.8 percent), and diabetes with nephropathy (13.0 percent) (Islam 2009). Diabetes is prevalent in slums and non-slums (table 2.1).

A study of diabetic patients registered in BIRDEM (Bangladesh Institute of Research and Rehabilitation in Diabetes, Endocrine and Metabolic Disorders) in Dhaka, found that within a few years of the onset of diabetes, 95 percent of young women from the lower socioeconomic classes were either divorced or deserted by their husbands, sometimes being left with one or two children (Mahtab and Chowdhury 2002). Another study found that 40 percent of people with diabetes cannot support themselves (Emneus et al. 2005).

The 2010 HIES found that 5.4 percent of the population suffered from diabetes, with wide variations by locality (3.4 percent in rural and 11.5 percent in urban populations) and gender (6.7 percent among males and 4.3 percent among females). The 2010 NCD Risk Factor Survey found that the proportion of adults (aged 25 years or over) who self-reported (documented) diabetes was 3.9 percent, with substantial variations by locality (figure 2.10).

NCD Risk Factors

NCDs such as CVDs, cancer, respiratory diseases, and diabetes are linked to a few common risk factors (figure 2.11).

Table 2.1   Diabetes Prevalence among Urban Men and Women, Aged 35 Years and Above, by Background Characteristics, Bangladesh, 2006

Percent

Background characteristics	Slum		Non-slum	
	Male	*Female*	*Male*	*Female*
Age				
<40	5.9	3.5	11.5	9.0
40–49	3.9	6.1	7.4	7.4
50–59	17.3	6.7	26.0	49.7
60–69	11.7	(11.6)	17.7	22.6
70+	(9.8)	(0.0)	24.5	(15.2)
Education level				
No education	5.2	5.9	3.2	13.7
Primary incomplete	6.8	1.8	7.4	6.7
Primary complete	3.9	(3.9)	9.3	20.1
Secondary incomplete	14.7	(4.2)	10.1	25.8
Secondary complete or higher	18.5	(18.1)	22.9	19.9
Household wealth quintile				
Poorest	3.3	1.9	(3.7)	(0.0)
2	5.7	2.2	2.0	(2.2)
3	6.5	8.0	6.0	3.8
4	14.6	9.0	12.4	12.9
Richest	(36.1)	(14.3)	21.5	24.9
Total	8.4	5.5	14.2	17.0

Source: NIPORT *et al.* 2008.

Figure 2.10   Diabetes Prevalence (Self-Reported) among Adults, Aged 25 Years and Above, by Locality and Gender, Bangladesh, 2010

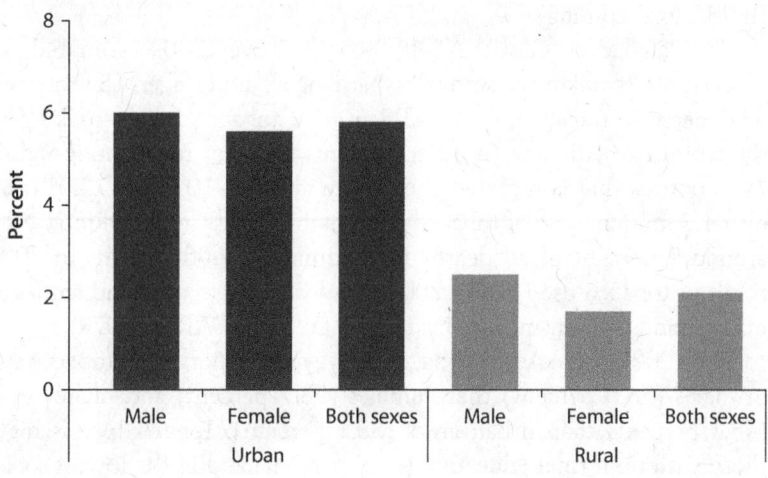

Source: WHO BD 2011.

Figure 2.11 Leading Risk Factors for Bangladesh, 2010 Estimates

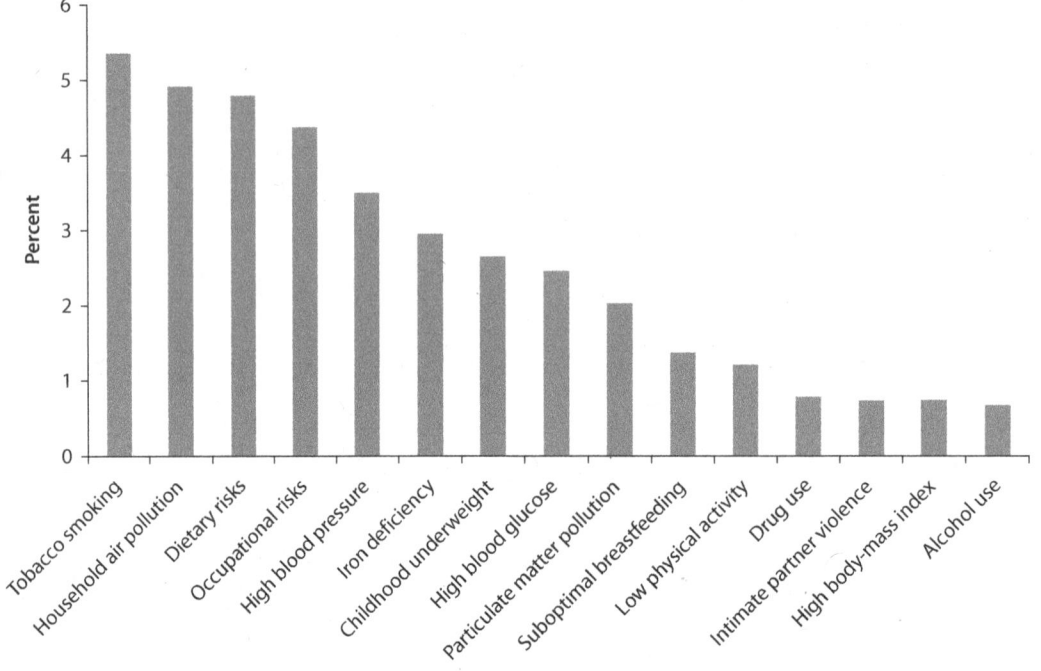

Source: IHME forthcoming.
Note: See appendix 1 for a detailed table.

Tobacco—Undermining the Health of Adults and Children, Draining Resources of the Poor

According to the WHO report on the Global Tobacco Epidemic, 2008, nearly two-thirds of the world's smokers live in 10 countries, of which one is Bangladesh (WHO 2008b). In 2010, tobacco smoking was the leading risk factor in Bangladesh and accounted for 5.4 percent of the total BOD or 2,779,870 DALYs (IHME forthcoming).

The Bangladesh Global Adult Tobacco Survey 2009 estimated that current tobacco use (smoking or smokeless) among all adults aged 15 years and over was 43.3 percent, translating into 41.3 million tobacco users—making Bangladesh the country with the most prevalent tobacco use among adults in the 14 countries that completed the survey in 2008–10 (WHO 2011a). There are over 1.2 million cases of tobacco-attributable illness in the country each year and around 9 percent of all deaths (an estimated 57,000 deaths in 2004) are the result of tobacco use (WHO 2007). Exposure to secondhand smoking kills tens of thousands of nonsmokers every year (WHO SEARO 2007a).

The 2009 Global Adult Tobacco Survey also reports that tobacco use is higher in males (58.0 percent) than females (28.7 percent) and higher in rural areas (45.1 percent) than urban areas (38.1 percent). Tobacco use is higher among those with no formal education (62.9 percent) and in the lowest socioeconomic quintiles (55.6 percent) (WHO BD 2009).

Figure 2.12 Tobacco Use among Adults, Aged 25 Years and Above, by Locality, Bangladesh, 2010

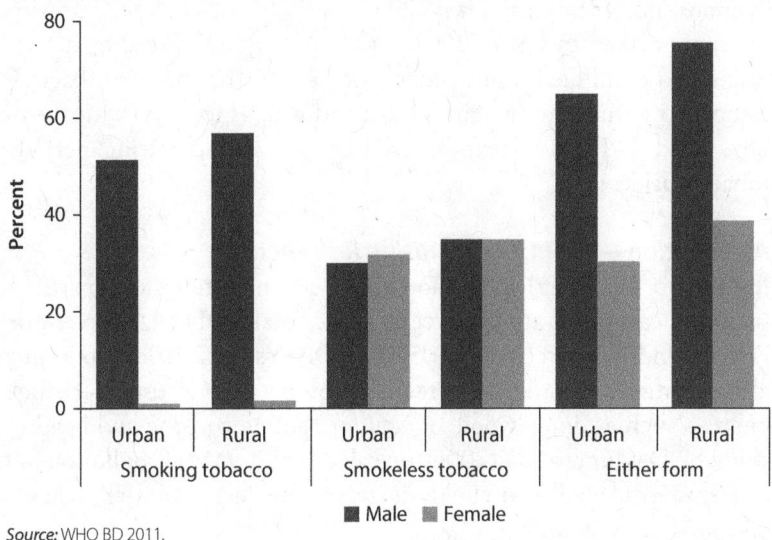

Source: WHO BD 2011.

The Bangladesh NCD Risk Factor Survey 2010 reports that 75 percent of rural males 25 years and older used tobacco compared with 65 percent of urban males; for women, the proportions are 39 and 30 percent, respectively (figure 2.12). This translates into 32.8 million people in Bangladesh (22.1 million males and 10.7 million females) who use any form of tobacco (WHO BD 2011).

Female rates of smoking are generally low (0.8 percent urban and 1.8 percent rural) but increase slightly with age. But Koehlmoos (2010) reports anecdotal evidence of potentially hidden rates of smoking among college women and the urban elite. Because of cultural norms against female smoking, women are more likely to partake of locally available smoke-free tobacco products, including *jarda* and *shada pata* (both dried tobacco leaves) (DGHS 2007). An increase in use of these products can be seen with age and from urban areas (22.5 percent) to rural areas (28.8 percent) (WHO BD 2009).

Tobacco use affects household food security and child health. Average cigarette spending per month among cigarette smokers was about $5.40 and among *bidi* smokers $1.90; total expenditure on cigarettes and *bidis* is 1.4 percent of gross domestic product (GDP) (WHO BD 2009). About 5 percent of household expenditure goes toward tobacco in the homes of smokers (WHO SEARO 2007a).

That more tobacco use occurs among lower socioeconomic groups is a common finding in Bangladesh-based tobacco studies (Choudhury *et al.* 2007; DGHS 2007). Poor families' scarce resources are spent on tobacco products instead of food, and can cause immediate harm to family members. For the poorest households in Bangladesh, among whom malnutrition is widespread, increasing tobacco prices may well shift much tobacco spending to food, significantly improving households' nutritional status—one report indicated that if poor people in Bangladesh did not smoke, 10.5 million fewer people would be malnourished (Efroymson *et al.* 2001).

Nonnemaker and Sur (2007) evaluated the relationship between tobacco prices and child health outcomes. They found that higher tobacco prices were associated with better height for age and weight for age (with the exception of boys aged 2–10, who experienced more wasting during periods of higher tobacco prices).

Air Pollution—The Insidious, Rising Risk Factor

IHME (forthcoming) puts household air pollution and particulate matter pollution combined at 6.9 percent of the total BOD (4.9 percent or 2,547,293 DALYs, and 2.0 percent or 1,054,738 DALYs) in 2010. Indoor air pollution is almost entirely ignored: 89 percent of the population uses solid fuels, including biomass such as dung, wood, or coal for routine cooking and heating. An earlier study by Dasgupta *et al.* (2006) revealed that indoor air pollution in the poorest and least-educated households is twice the levels of the richest and better educated households.

Urban air quality continues to deteriorate due to pollution by automobiles and industries. Reducing exposure to urban air pollution by 20–80 percent could save 1,200–3,500 lives annually and avoid 80–230 million cases of disease (World Bank 2006).

Diet and Nutrition—Too Much of the Wrong Fats and Salt, but Too Few Vegetables and Fruits

Poor nutrition habits and lack of awareness of healthy diets result in diets rich in saturated fats, salt, and refined carbohydrates, which may increase the risk of NCDs, particularly CVD and diabetes. Dietary risks were the third leading risk factor in 2010 and accounted for 4.8 percent or 2,484,757 DALYs (IHME forthcoming). Countries developing economically exhibit a nutrition transition characterized by an increase in consumption of fats and simple sugars coupled with a decrease in the intake of fruits and vegetables. The nutrition transition under way in many Asian countries is characterized by moving from the traditional diets that are high in carbohydrates and low in fat, to one higher in fat and lower in complex carbohydrates. In addition, macronutrients such as edible oils play an important role in increasing the risk of NCDs. For example, transfats and saturated fatty acids add to the risk for coronary heart diseases.

The 2010 HIES estimated per capita edible oil consumption (all types) increased to 20.5 grams in 2010 from 16.5 grams in 2000. It also found that per capita oil consumption is much higher in urban areas (26.6 grams per day) than in rural areas (18.3 grams per day). However, it constitutes only 7.9 percent of daily per capita calorie intake, which is much lower than the dietary recommendations of WHO and the Food and Agriculture Organization of the United Nations (Irz, Shankar, and Srinivasan 2003).

Table 2.2 Per Capita Edible Oil Consumption in Bangladesh
Grams per day

Demographics	Rural	Urban	Total
Age[a] (year)			
1–3	2	2.5	2.1
4–6	4	6.5	4.5
7–9	4.8	7.8	5.4
Gender[b]			
Female	7.1	13.4	8.4
Male	10	20.3	12.1

Source: Jahan and Hossain 1998.
a. For children aged 1–9 years.
b. For all ages.

An earlier study on edible oil consumption (all types) by age and gender found that per capita consumption is higher for children of older age groups and significantly higher (about 45 percent) for men than women (table 2.2). The two consumption characteristics apply to rural and urban areas (Jahan and Hossain 1998). During 1999–2002, a rapid increase in per capita consumption of soybean oil and palm oil was documented (MOST 2004).

The Bangladesh NCD Risk Factor Survey 2010 documented that 60 million people (30.8 million men and 29.2 million women) reported low vegetable and fruit intake (defined as fewer than five servings a day) (WHO BD 2011).

High salt intake is an important contributing factor for high blood pressure. A small study from urban and rural populations documented high consumption of salt, with an average 24-hour salt intake of 17 grams per day (Choudhury *et al.* 2010). Another report documented pilot studies using spot urine samples, which indicated that salt intake among the population is very high, reaching 16–18 grams per day (rural and urban), and that much salt is added at table (WHO 2010).

High Blood Pressure (Hypertension)—An Alarming Risk Factor

A nonsystematic review conducted by Zaman and Rouf (1999) included three articles, which employed nonstandard high blood pressure definitions and were limited to populations in Dhaka during 1979–94. Because of heterogeneity and a lack of appropriate categorization in the primary studies, the review was inconclusive on the prevalence of high blood pressure (or hypertension) in Bangladesh and recommended that a large study on the risk factor be undertaken.

Studies with relatively small sample sizes (240 urban and rural), such as the India–Bangladesh study conducted by the Hypertension Study Group in 2001, found an overall hypertension rate of 65 percent in populations over 60 years of age. They have given way in recent years to more rigorously designed studies with sample sizes greater than 2,000 (Razzaque *et al.* 2009; Sayeed *et al.* 2002). The later studies found lack of physical activity, overweight, age, and higher socioeconomic status positively associated with higher levels of hypertension or high blood pressure (or both) (Razzaque *et al.* 2011). Although the WHO STEP-wise approach to surveillance (STEPS) methodology has been applied in numerous studies conducted in Bangladesh by the Bangladesh Rural Advancement Committee (BRAC), International Centre for Diarrhoeal Disease Research, Bangladesh (ICDDR,B), and other agencies, Bangladesh did not report prevalence of raised blood pressure nor prevalence of known hypertension and its treatment in WHO regional reports (WHO SEARO 2007b). Although there is no representative sample of high blood pressure (or hypertension) in Bangladesh, hypertensive patients attending clinics have been used to test interventions for tobacco cessation and to capture the clustering of metabolic factors (Ahmed, Choudhury, and Zaman 2007; Siddique *et al.* 2008).

The 2006 Bangladesh Urban Health Survey looked at high blood pressure/hypertension (using a single blood pressure reading and self-reported medication use for hypertension in adults aged 35 years and over) in slum and non-slum areas of the six largest city corporations in Bangladesh (Dhaka, Chittagong, Khulna, Rajshahi, Barisal, and Sylhet). The survey found that 25 percent of slum-dwelling and 38 percent of non-slum-dwelling women had hypertension. Among men, 18 percent were hypertensive in the slums and 25 percent in the non-slum areas. Hypertension increased with age, wealth quintile, and education. Among non-slum women aged 60–69, 64.3 percent had hypertension compared with 37.1 percent of slum women of the same age (NIPORT *et al.* 2008).

The Bangladesh NCD Risk Factor Survey 2010 reported that 17.9 percent of adults (18.5 percent males and 17.3 percent females) aged 25 years or more were hypertensive, defined as having raised blood pressure of 140/90 mmHg or higher (or currently on medication), which translated into 12 million people in total. Figure 2.13 shows the prevalence by locality and gender. The study also found that 11.6 million people (17.6 percent of the population aged 25 years or

Figure 2.13 Prevalence of High Blood Pressure/Hypertension (BP ≥ 140/90 mmHg or on Medication) among Adults Aged 25 Years or More by Locality and Gender, Bangladesh, 2010

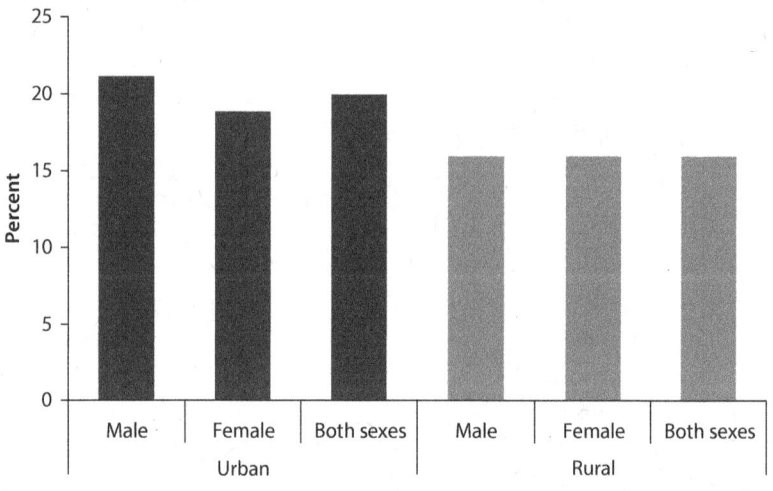

Source: WHO BD 2011.

more) were overweight, out of whom 6.7 million were female (21.6 percent), and 13 million (21.7 percent) had large waist circumference (2.5 million men and 10.5 million women), which is defined as a circumference of more than 94 cm for men and more than 80 cm for women (WHO BD 2011). High blood pressure accounted for 3.5 percent of the total BOD in 2010 (1,817,797 DALYs) (IHME forthcoming).

Malnutrition and Low Birth Weight—An Early Double Burden

The risk of NCDs starts during gestation and infancy, accumulates from early childhood, and is influenced by factors acting in all stages of the life span (Aboderin *et al.* 2001). Several studies have shown that malnourished women tend to deliver low-birth-weight babies who are more likely to have stunted growth, cognitive impairment, poor school performance, fewer years of schooling, and reduced productivity, which all increase the probability of developing CVDs and hypertension (Barker *et al.* 1989; Johansson *et al.* 2005).

In childhood, poor dietary habits and overnutrition may lead to childhood obesity, which increases the propensity for developing NCDs in adulthood. Additionally, poverty, poor education, lack of access to basic amenities such as clean water, and lack of access to information exacerbate matters and make large segments of the population prone to acquiring NCDs in the later stages of life. This combined, increased risk of NCDs results from both biological mechanisms and social determinants. They are interrelated and have a transgenerational impact (figure 2.14).

Figure 2.14 Low Birth Weight and the Transgenerational Effect in Increasing the Risk of NCDs

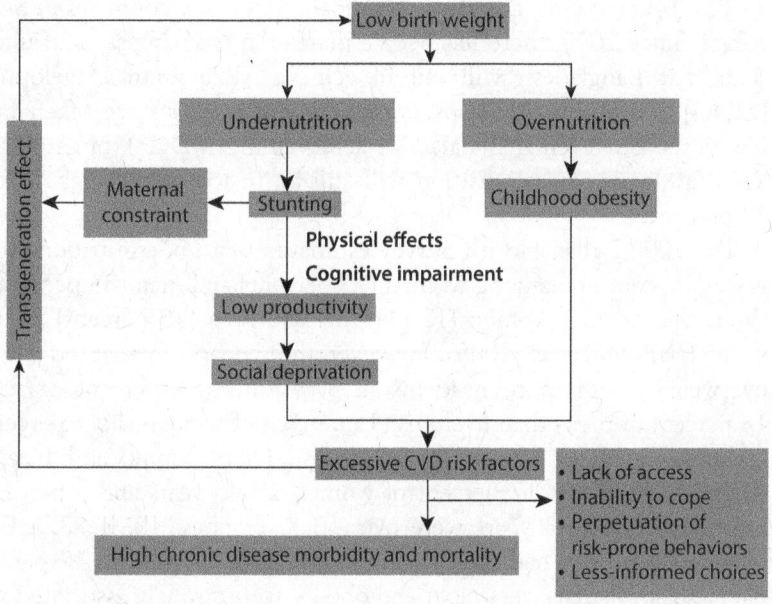

Sources: Based on Aboderin *et al.* 2001; Smith 2007.

In order to test Barker's hypothesis (Barker 1992; Barker and Clark 1997)[4] and to examine the association between prenatal exposure to undernutrition during the Bangladesh famine of 1974–75, a case control study was conducted in a subsample of the Matlab Health and Demographic Surveillance System population that looked for abnormalities of glucose and lipid metabolism in early adulthood (27–31 years of age). The results suggested that prenatal exposure to undernutrition is associated with elevated risk of IGT in young adults (Alam et al. 2006).

In Bangladesh, rates of low birth weight are among the highest in the world (UNICEF/WHO 2004). The National Low Birth Weight Survey of Bangladesh 2003–04 found a prevalence of 36 percent (UNICEF/BBS 2005). Multivariate analysis revealed that maternal nutrition and pregnancy-related factors were important predictors of low birth weight. Controlling for the independent effects of other covariates, maternal body mass index (BMI) and height were powerful predictors of low birth weight. Cultural beliefs in rural areas promote that pregnant women should limit their weight gain (and thus calorific intake) during pregnancy with the idea that a smaller fetus will lead to an easier and safer birth. The 2003–04 survey also found that girls in all settings were more likely to be low birth weight than boys (37.9 versus 33.3 percent) and that rural newborns were more likely to be low birth weight than their urban counterparts (36.7 versus 20.0 percent).

Bangladesh also has one of the highest proportions of undernourished people in the world. More than 40 percent of children under five are either moderately underweight (weight-for-age <–2 standard deviations [SD]) or moderately stunted (height-for-age <–2 SD) or both (NIPORT et al. 2009). About 17 percent of under-five children are moderately wasted (weight-for-height <–2 SD). These rates are much higher than in many countries in Sub-Saharan Africa. Since 2000, there has been a plateau in reducing rates of underweight, such that Bangladesh will fail to achieve Millennium Development Goal (MDG) 1 if the trend is sustained and unless efforts are taken in the next few years. But even if Bangladesh achieves the MDG 1 target for nutrition, the prevalence of malnutrition will still be unacceptably high, at more than 33 percent.

The 2006 Urban Health Survey estimated that undernutrition (BMI <18.5) was more common among women (27 percent) and men (35 percent) in urban slums than among women (13 percent) and men (19 percent) in urban non-slums (NIPORT et al. 2008). However, the scenario is reversed for obesity or overweight, with more residents in non-slums (34 percent of women and 18 percent of men) than in slums (15 percent of women and 7 percent of men) classified as obese. The 2011 Bangladesh Demographic and Health Survey (BDHS) found that 17 percent of women 15–49 years and 7 percent of ever-married men 15–34 years were overweight or obese (BMI >25). From 2007, overweight/obesity had increased by nearly half, from 12 to 17 percent. These data also show that overweight and obesity were strongly associated with socio-economic status (figure 2.15).

Figure 2.15 Overweight and Obesity Status among Males and Females, Bangladesh, 2011

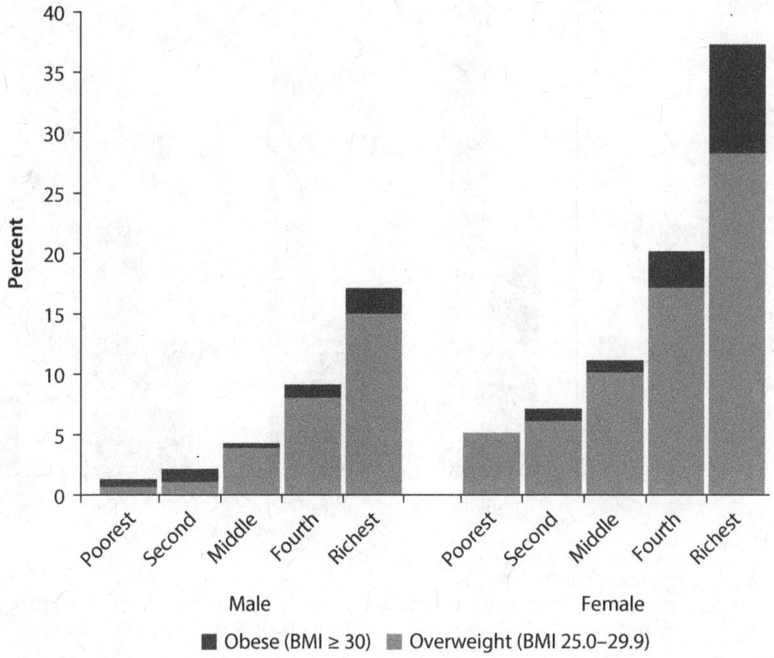

Source: NIPORT et al. 2012.
Note: BMI = body mass index.

Physical Activity—Lower Rates among Women

A multicenter cross-sectional study of chronic NCD risk factors conducted in nine rural Health and Demographic Surveillance System sites in five Asian countries (including four sites in Bangladesh) in 2008 showed the age-adjusted prevalence of physical inactivity to range, among men, from 12 to 35 percent and among women, from 21 to 65 percent (figure 2.16). Physical inactivity was more prevalent among men and women in the youngest (25–34 years) and oldest (55–64 years) age groups (Ng et al. 2009).

The Bangladesh NCD Risk Factor Survey 2010 reported that 16.1 million people have low physical activity, defined as less than 600 MET (metabolic equivalents)—3.3 million men and 12.8 million women (WHO BD 2011).

Alcohol Consumption and Substance Abuse—Small but Seemingly Rising

The consumption of alcohol in Bangladesh is strictly prohibited both socially and by most religions. However, information from law enforcement authorities, treatment providers, and other sources indicates that alcohol abuse is increasing. Although the problem is more serious in urban areas (probably due to easy accessibility of alcoholic beverages), there are indications that it is emerging at an increasing rate in rural areas. Nationally, alcohol consumption in 2003 was below 0.5 liters per capita (WHO 2004). However, the latest report by WHO estimated that the average per capita consumption by the Bangladeshi population aged 15

Figure 2.16 Prevalence of Physical Inactivity in Four Sites in Bangladesh

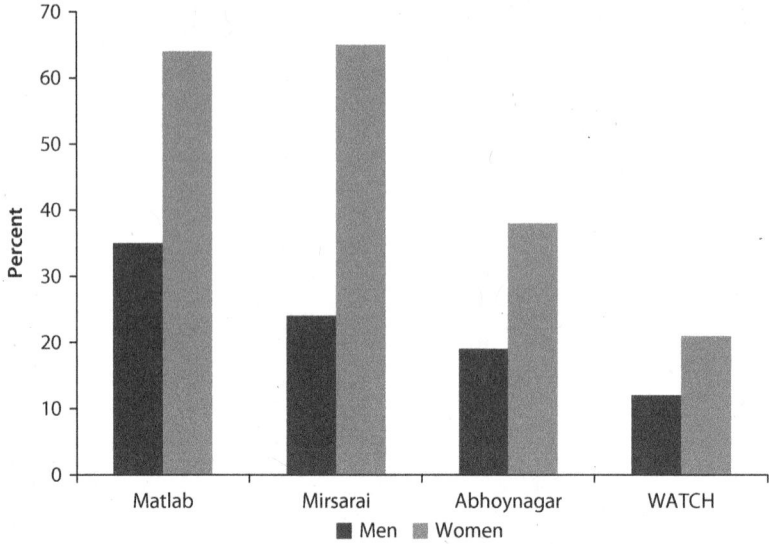

Source: Ng *et al.* 2009.
Note: The WATCH site is maintained by Bangladesh Rural Advancement Committee and covers a population of about 90,000 in 85 villages in 10 rural regions and 4 urban clusters in one large city.

and above during 2003–05 to be 0.2 liters of pure alcohol, and among the drinkers the average was 4.47 (for males 4.59 liters and for females 2.98 liters). The report also estimated that among adults aged 15 years or more in 2003, the proportion of heavy episodic drinkers was 7.5 percent among males and 3.3 percent among females (WHO 2011b).

Alcohol is produced by some pharmaceutical industries in Bangladesh. Moreover, some crude forms are produced and used by the poor, usually by fermenting boiled rice, sugarcane, and molasses. Although no systematic assessment has been undertaken to establish the prevalence and patterns of substance abuse, different government and nongovernment drug addiction and treatment centers, as well as various journals and studies, report increasing drug-related crimes in the country (WHO 2004). The younger generation in Bangladesh, especially students, are most vulnerable to substance abuse (WHO 2004).

At least 90 Bangladeshis died in 1998, including 70 in Gaibandha district, after consuming illegal homemade alcohol. In the following year, there was an incident of alcohol poisoning in the northeastern town of Narsingdi (about 50 miles from Dhaka), where 96 people reportedly died and more than 100 were hospitalized as a result of drinking illegal homemade liquor. A 1995 study of 30 male multiple drug users (aged 20 years and above) found that alcohol was one of the most frequently used drugs (50 percent of the sample reported use of alcohol prior to the interview) (Ahmed and Ara 2001).

The Bangladesh NCD Risk Factor Survey 2010 reported that 94.4 percent of the population aged 25 years and over were lifetime abstainers, and 0.9 percent had consumed alcohol (1.5 percent males and 0.1 percent females) in the preceding months. However, the study found that the majority (66.7 percent) of current drinkers were involved in binge drinking (five or more standard drinks for men, and four or more for women) (WHO BD 2011).

Among the urban population, the proportions of men reporting "ever use" of drugs and alcohol were identical across slum and non-slum areas of city corporations (around 12 percent), and notably lower than among men in district municipalities (17.3 percent) (NIPORT *et al.* 2008). A study of the homeless in Dhaka revealed that 69 percent of men reported using some type of illegal drug during the previous year; 73 percent of them had smoked marijuana and 12 percent had used heroine (Koehlmoos *et al.* 2009). A study by the World Bank found that nearly one in every 10 street children aged 11–19 years in major metropolitan cities had ever consumed alcohol (Mahmud, Ahsan, and Claeson 2011).

In addition to the above leading risk factors, excessive arsenic poisoning in drinking water is a major public health threat (box 2.3).

Economic and Social Impact

NCDs can hold back economic development and efforts to reduce poverty in low-income countries. They may reduce per capita income through ripple effects caused by a reduced labor force and lower productivity, increased dependency ratio, reduced access to factors of production, increased consumption, reduced savings, and decreased investment in physical capital (figure 2.17).

Box 2.3 Arsenic—Still a Major Public Health Threat

Described by Smith, Lingas, and Rahman (2000) as "the largest mass poisoning of a population in history," excessive arsenic in drinking water is a unique risk factor for NCDs in Bangladesh and parts of West Bengal where arsenic levels are naturally high. Tubewells, which were introduced during the 1970s and 1980s to gather water free of bacteria and pesticides, literally tap into the surface level that contains the arsenic. For short exposure (generally revealed through skin lesions or darkening), the cure is merely to abstain from arsenic-laced water; however, for those with long-term exposure, there is an increased risk of hypertension; diabetes (due to insulin deficiency); and skin, lung, bladder, and kidney cancer (Bates, Smith, and Hopenhayn-Rich 1992; Smith *et al.* 1992).

Of 4.7 million tubewells in Bangladesh, 1.7 million were found to contain an unacceptable level of contamination (that is, an arsenic level of more than 50 parts per billion) (UNICEF 2008). Approximately 20 million people in Bangladesh are exposed to this risk factor (UNICEF 2008). Early efforts focused on diagnosing impact through the observation of skin lesions; however, it is hypothesized that the greatest morbidity impact from arsenic exposure will be from lung cancer (Kaufmann *et al.* 2002).

Other than arsenic, contamination of water reservoirs with pesticides remains a widespread problem in many countries of the region, including Bangladesh, and it has been linked to a higher incidence of cancer, birth defects, and infertility (Khan *et al.* 2003).

Figure 2.17 The Macroeconomic Effects of NCDs

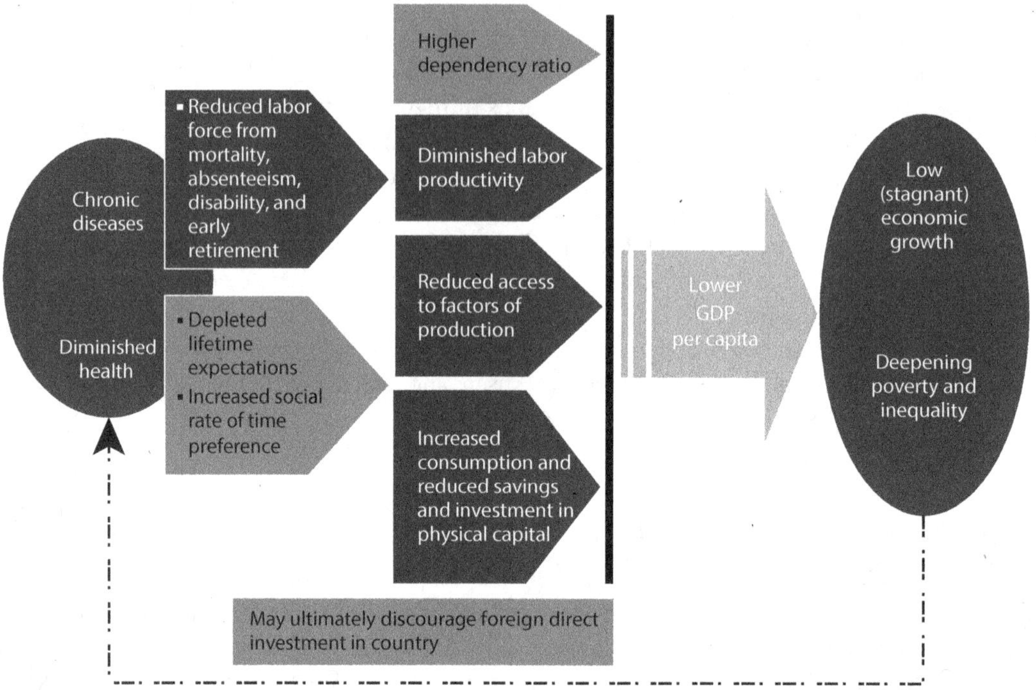

Source: Abegunde and Stanciole 2006.
Note: GDP = gross domestic product; NCDs = noncommunicable diseases.

Economic Burden—Higher on the Poor

Although empirical evidence is scant for South Asia, projections from a few years ago suggested that over the next 10 years, deaths from heart disease, stroke, and diabetes may have been set to lower GDP in India and Pakistan by 1 percent (WHO 2005). In Sri Lanka, where life expectancy has increased the most in the region, chronic illness is an important cause of withdrawal from the labor market (World Bank 2008).

In Bangladesh, there are very few studies of the economic impact of NCDs. One WHO study found that tobacco was a major risk factor and cost the economy about $44 million annually (WHO SEARO 2007a). Another study estimated that each episode of smoking-related illness cost up to $66, which is equivalent to two or three months of an average income (Ali, Rahman, and Rahman 2003). For low-income groups, direct costs associated with diabetic care could drain up to 24.5 percent of annual household income (Shobhana *et al.* 2000).

Spending on the risk factors for NCDs and on managing these disorders can also undermine families' financial status—Bangladeshi smokers spend on average more than twice as much on cigarettes as on health, education, housing, and clothing (Efroymson *et al.* 2001). Treatment for diabetes can cost 6–12 months' wages ($160 a year) (Kibriya *et al.* 1999). Another study showed that about half of rural poor households in Bangladesh had not been poor before a traffic accident (Aeron-Thomas *et al.* 2004). The total annual cost of road traffic accidents is estimated at $230 million a year (DGHS 2007).

IDF has estimated the mean diabetes-related expenditure for Bangladesh at $28 per person a year (IDF 2012). Given the current estimated size of the country's diabetic population (NIPORT *et al.* 2013), nearly $150 million would be required every year. This figure could well rise to $262 million in a short time, as one-third of pre-diabetics are likely to convert into diabetics (Wang *et al.* 2010). This higher figure is equivalent to 24 percent of the total budget of the Ministry of Health and Family Welfare (MOHFW) in FY2010/11 (Government of Bangladesh 2011).

In brief, the NCD epidemic has a huge direct impact on financial vulnerability, particularly for the poor, and an indirect impact on the economy. Policy makers should consider both these factors when formulating NCD-related policies, aided by considering the social determinants of NCDs.

Social Determinants

Social determinants play an important role in health, and the degree of social disadvantage and poverty within countries is closely linked to dramatic health differences (CSDH 2008). These inequities arise because of the circumstances in which people grow, live, work, and age, and because of the systems put in place to deal with health and illness. These circumstances in turn are shaped by political, social, and economic forces. In addition, the relationship between NCDs and poverty is bidirectional, through social determinants (figure 2.18).

In developed countries, the poor and disadvantaged experience a larger burden of risk factors and NCDs than the rich. In South Asia, the burden may currently be greater in the rich, but it is set to shift in line with the developed country experience and be concentrated among the poor. Risk factors such as

Figure 2.18 Social Determinants, NCDs, and Their Relationship to Poverty

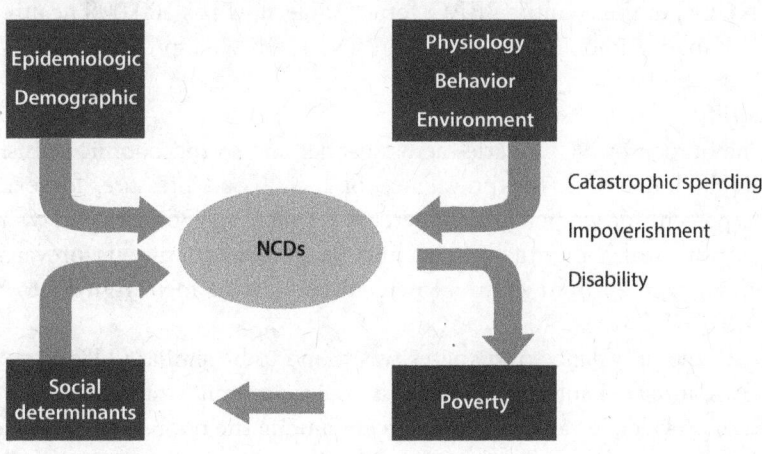

Source: Engelgau *et al.* 2011.
Note: NCDs = noncommunicable diseases.

tobacco use are already more common among the poor. Addressing social determinants requires not only health policies that are sensitive to the situation but also efforts from many non-health sectors, especially education and social protection. Most of the development agenda—economic opportunities; the distribution of power, money, and resources; and living conditions—influence social determinants.

The major social development strides that Bangladesh has made may be explained by four main factors (*The Economist* 2012). First, women's social empowerment through family planning and education has improved their status in the community. In 1975, 8 percent of women of child-bearing age were using contraception (or had partners who were); in 2010, the rate was over 60 percent. In giving women better health and more autonomy, family planning was one of a number of factors that improved their lot, and by so doing did much to reduce poverty. The spread of primary education, particularly for girls, was one of the others (the government has been better than many at helping women this way); the proportion of girls who are schooled has increased much more than the proportion of boys.

Second, Bangladesh managed to restrain the fall in rural household incomes that usually increases extreme poverty in developing countries. Between 1971 and 2010, the rice harvest more than trebled, though the area under cultivation increased by less than 10 percent. For the last few years, the country, once supposedly doomed to dependence on food aid, has been a small exporter of rice.

Third, villages have found resources from beyond agriculture—and, indeed, beyond Bangladesh. Around 6 million Bangladeshis work abroad, mostly in the Middle East, and they remit a larger share of the national income than any other big country gets from migrants. In the year ending June 2012, they sent back $13 billion, about 14 percent of national income—more than all the government's social-protection programs put together. The majority of migrant workers send their remittances back to family members in the village they came from.

Fourth is the extraordinary role played by nongovernmental organizations (NGOs) in the country. BRAC, for example, now has 100,000 health volunteers with mobile phones (mobile-phone coverage is widespread in Bangladesh).

Equity

The burden of NCDs varies across gender and socioeconomic status. The 2011 BDHS found that the prevalence of high blood pressure, for example, was 32 percent for women and 19 percent for men, age 35 years and over. From the poorest wealth quintile to the highest wealth quintile, its prevalence varied among women from 25 to 44 percent and among men from 13 to 30 percent (NIPORT 2013).

While prevalence of diabetes was found to be similar (11 percent) for both sexes, it varied substantially across socioeconomic strata. For women 35 and over, prevalence varied from 7 percent among the poorest to 21 percent among the richest; for men, the corresponding figures were 8 and 20 percent (NIPORT 2013).

The 2006 Bangladesh Urban Health Survey showed that, for adult men, household wealth quintile held the greatest difference, such that the richest households in non-slum areas reported 28.5 percent with high blood pressure, versus 6.0 percent for the lowest wealth quintile. The extreme was greater in the slum areas, where 31.2 percent of men in the highest quintile had high blood pressure versus 13.0 percent in the lowest. For females, the difference for high blood pressure is less, despite higher prevalence (in slums: 22.3 percent with high blood pressure in the poorest quintile versus 47.5 percent in the richest quintile; in non-slums: 21.5 versus 42.8 percent, respectively) (NIPORT *et al.* 2008).

The prevalence of diabetes among males and females aged 35 and above differs substantially by socioeconomic status. In non-slums, no women from the poorest quintile reported having diabetes, while exactly one in every four women from the richest quintile had diabetes. For males living in urban non-slums, this difference is 3.7 versus 21.5 percent, respectively (NIPORT *et al.* 2008).

The prevalence of serious injury among males and females aged 15–59 also worsens with decreasing socioeconomic status. The worst was for men living in slums: 12.3 percent of the poorest quintile experienced a serious injury in the previous year compared with 1.5 percent of the richest quintile. For females in urban non-slums, 10.6 percent of the poorest quintile experienced a serious injury in the previous year compared with 4.6 percent of the richest quintile (NIPORT *et al.* 2008).

Notes

1. Figures in this section use crude (not age standardized) estimates to reflect the actual population burden, unlike figure 1.4. This accounts for the difference in the estimates between the two sections.

2. Conventionally, major NCDs include heart disease, stroke, diabetes, cancer, and chronic respiratory diseases (DGHS 2007).

3. Type 1 diabetes is most commonly found in youth and younger adults, and treatment requires insulin. Type 2 is most commonly found in mature adults, and initial treatment usually does not require insulin—although long-term cases typically need insulin.

4. Barker's hypothesis postulates that reduced fetal growth is strongly associated with a number of chronic conditions in later life.

References

Abegunde, D., and A. Stanciole. 2006. "An Estimation of the Economic Impact of Chronic Noncommunicable Diseases in Selected Countries." Working Paper, World Health Organization, Geneva, Switzerland.

Abegunde, D., C. Mathers, T. Adam, M. Ortegon, and K. Strong. 2007. "The Burden and Costs of Chronic Diseases in Low-income and Middle-income Countries." *The Lancet* 370: 1929–38.

Aboderin, I., A. Kalache, Y. Ben-Shlomo, J. Lynch, C. Yajnik, D. Kuh, and D. Yach. 2001. *Life Course Perspectives on Coronary Heart Disease, Stroke and Diabetes: Key Issues and Implications for Policy and Research*. Geneva, Switzerland: World Health Organization.

Aeron-Thomas, A., G. Jacobs, B. Sexton, G. Gururaj, and F. Rahman. 2004. "The Involvement and Impact of Road Crashes on the Poor: Bangladesh and India Case Studies." Project report for Global Road Safety Partnership, Geneva, Switzerland. http://www.grsproadsafety.org/themes/default/pdfs/The%20Poor-_final %20final%20report.pdf.

Ahmed, S. K., and N. Ara. 2001. "An Exploratory Study of Buprenorphine Use in Bangladesh: A Note." *Substance Use and Misuse* 36 (8): 1071–83.

Ahmed, J., S. R. Choudhury, and M. M. Zaman. 2007. "Tobacco Cessation in a Rural Health Center of Bangladesh." Paper presented at the National Conference on Cardiovascular Diseases, Dhaka, December 1–2.

Alam, D. S., M. Yunus, L. Ali, and A. K. Saha. 2006. "Prenatal Exposure to Undernutrition and Glucose and Lipid Metabolism in Young Adults in Rural Matlab, Bangladesh." Abstract in DOHaD Conference, Utrecht, September 13–16.

Ali, Z., A. Rahman, and T. Rahman. 2003. "Appetite for Nicotine: An Economic Analysis of Tobacco Control in Bangladesh." HNP Discussion Paper Series, Economics of Tobacco Control Paper 16, World Bank, Washington, DC.

Barker, D. J. 1992. "The Fetal Origins of Diseases of Old Age." *European Journal of Clinical Nutrition* 46 (Suppl 3): S3–9.

Barker, D. J., and P. M. Clark. 1997. "Fetal Undernutrition and Disease in Later Life." *Reviews of Reproduction* 2 (2): 105–12.

Barker D. J., C. Osmond, P. D. Winter, B. Margetts, and S. J. Simmonds. 1989. "Weight in Infancy and Death from Ischaemic Heart Disease." *The Lancet* 334 (8663): 577–80.

Bates, M. N., A. H. Smith, and C. Hopenhayn-Rich C. 1992. "Arsenic Ingestion and Internal Cancers: A Review." *American Journal of Epidemiology* 135 (5): 462–76.

BBS (Bangladesh Bureau of Statistics). 2011a. *Report on Sample Vital Registration System 2010*. Dhaka.

———. 2011b. *Preliminary Report on Household Income and Expenditure Survey 2010*. Dhaka.

Boutayeb, A., and S. Boutayeb. 2005. "The Burden of Noncommunicable Diseases in Developing Countries." *International Journal for Equity in Health* 4: 2. doi: 10.1186/1475-9276-4-2.

Cancer Care Program Bangladesh. 2010. http://www.cancercareprogram.org/v2/hpv.html.

Celli, B. R., R. J. Halbert, S. Isonaka, and B. Schau. 2003. "Population Impact of Different Definitions of Airway Obstruction." *European Respiratory Journal* 22: 268–73.

Choudhury, S., J. Ahmed, M. Zaman, M. Sobhan, and A. Hussain. 2011. "Burden of Stroke and its Related Disabilities in a Rural Community of Bangladesh." *Journal of Epidemiology & Community Health* 65 (Suppl 1): A231.

Choudhury, K., S. M. A. Hanifi, S. S. Mahmood, and A. Bhuiya. 2007. "Sociodemographic Characteristics of Tobacco Consumers in a Rural Area of Bangladesh." *Journal of Health, Population and Nutrition* 25 (4): 456–64.

Choudhury, S., F. Tabassum, J. Ahmed, M. Zaman, A. Rouf, R. Khandaker, and A. Malik. 2010. "Daily Salt Intake Estimated from Urinary Excretion of Sodium in a Bangladeshi Population." Paper presented at World Congress of Cardiology, Beijing, June 16–19.

Choudhury, S., M. Zaman, J. Ahmed, M. Sobhan, T. Haque, and A. Malik. 2006. "Prevalence of Rheumatic Fever and Rheumatic Heart Disease in a Rural Population of Bangladesh." Paper presented at the World Congress of Cardiology, Barcelona, Spain, September 2–6.

CACB (Committee on the Aetiology of Chronic Bronchitis). 1965. "Definition and Classification of Chronic Bronchitis for Clinical and Epidemiological Purposes: A Report to the Medical Research Council by Their Committee on the Aetiology of Chronic Bronchitis." *Lancet* 1 (7389): 775–9.

CSDH (Commission on Social Determinants of Health). 2008. *Closing the Gap in a Generation: Health Equity through Action on the Social Determinants of Health*. Final report, World Health Organization, Geneva, Switzerland.

Dasgupta, S., M. Huq, M. Khaliquzzaman, K. Pandey, and D. Wheeler. 2006. "Who Suffers from Indoor Air Pollution? Evidence from Bangladesh." *Health Policy and Planning* 21 (6): 444–58.

DGHS (Directorate General of Health Services), MOHFW (Ministry of Health and Family Welfare). 2007. *Strategic Plan for Surveillance and Prevention of Non-Communicable Diseases in Bangladesh 2007–2010*. Dhaka: DGHS, MOHFW.

———. 2008. *National Cancer Control Strategy and Plan of Action 2009–2015*. Dhaka: MOHFW.

The Economist 2012. "Bangladesh and Development: The Path through the Fields." London, November 3.

Efroymson, D., S. Ahmed, J. Townsend, S. Alam, A.Dey, R. Saha, B. Dhar, A. Sujon, K. Ahmed, and O. Rahman. 2001. "Hungry for Tobacco: An Analysis of the Economic Impact of Tobacco Consumption on the Poor in Bangladesh." *Tobacco Control* 10 (3): 212–17.

Emneus, M., S. Bjork, T. Christiansen, and A. Green. 2005. "The Societal Impact of Diabetes Mellitus and Diabetes Care: A Case Study from Bangladesh, Year 2001." Proceedings of the 9th Global Forum, Mumbai, September 11–16.

Engelgau, M. M., S. El-Saharty, P. Kudesia, V. Rajan, S. Rosenhouse, and K. Okamoto. 2011. *Capitalizing on the Demographic Transition: Tackling Noncommunicable Diseases in South Asia*. Washington, DC: World Bank.

Government of Bangladesh. 2011. *Bangladesh Economic Review 2011*. Dhaka: Ministry of Finance.

Goyal, A., and S. Yusuf. 2006. "The Burden of Cardiovascular Disease in the Indian Subcontinent." *Indian Journal of Medical Research* 124 (September): 235–44.

Halbert, R. J., S. Isonaka, D. George, and A. Iqbal. 2003. "Interpreting COPD Prevalence Estimates. What is the True Burden of Disease?" *Chest* 123 (5): 1684–92.

Hussain, A., M. A. Rahim, A. K. Azad Khan, S. M. K. Ali, and S. Vaaler. 2005. "Type 2 Diabetes in Rural and Urban Population: Diverse Prevalence and Associated Risk Factors in Bangladesh." *Diabetic Medicine* 22 (7): 931– 36.

ICMH, DGHS, TASC, and UNICEF (Institute of Child and Mother Health, Directorate General of Health Services, The Alliance for Safe Children, and United Nations Children's Fund). 2005. *Bangladesh Health and Injuries Survey: Key Findings on Child Injury.* Dhaka: UNICEF. http://www.tasc-gcipf.org/downloads/Key%20Findings%20-%20BHIS.pdf

IDF (International Diabetes Federation). 2006a. *Diabetes Atlas*. Third Edition. Brussels: IDF.

————. 2006b. "Diabetic Association of Bangladesh Supports Unite for Diabetes." http://www.world-diabetesday.org/node/2918.

————. 2012. "IDF Diabetic Atlas: Country Summary Tables." https://www.idf.org/sites/default/files/5E_IDFAtlasPoster_2012_EN.pdf.

IHME (Institute for Health Metrics and Evaluation). Forthcoming. *Global Burden of Disease Study 2010. Bangladesh Results by Cause 1990–2010.* Seattle, WA.

Irz, X., B. Shankar, and C. S. Srinivasan. 2003. "Dietary Recommendations in the Report of a Joint WHO/FAO Expert Consultation on Diet, Nutrition and the Prevention of Chronic Diseases: Potential Impact on Consumption, Production and Trade of Selected Food Products." WHO Technical Report Series 916. http://www.hubrural.org/IMG/pdf/fao_who_report_diet.pdf

Islam, M. Z. 2009. "Disability Burden of Diabetes Mellitus and its Complications." *Journal of Medicine* 10 (Suppl 1): 22–6.

Jahan, K., and M. Hossain. 1998. *Nature and Extent of Malnutrition in Bangladesh: Bangladesh National Nutrition Survey, 1995–96.* Dhaka: Institute of Nutrition and Food Science, University of Dhaka.

Johansson, S., A. Iliadou, N. Bergvall, T. Tuvemo, M. Norman, and S. Cnattingius. 2005. "Risk of High Blood Pressure among Young Men Increases with the Degree of Immaturity at Birth." *Circulation* 112: 3430–36.

Kabiruzzaman, M. 2007. "Heart Failure: Incidence, Prevalence and Mortality—NHFH&RI Perspective." Paper presented at the National Heart Conference on Cardiovascular Diseases, Dhaka, December 1–2.

Kabiruzzaman, M., F. N. Malik, N. Ahmed, M. Badiuzzaman, S. R. Choudhury, T. Haque, H. Rahman, M. N. Ahmed, D. Banik, M. A. M. Khan, A. K. Dutta, S. Sayeed, R. K. Khandaker, and A. Malik. 2010. "Burden of Heart Failure Patients in a Tertiary Level Cardiac Hospital." *Journal of Bangladesh College of Physicians and Surgeons* 28 (1): 24–9.

Kaufmann, R., B. Sorensen, M. Rahman, P. K. Streatfield, L. A. Persson, L. Ake, and S. S. Gopalan. 2002. *Addressing the Public Health Crisis Caused by Arsenic Contamination of Drinking Water in Bangladesh.* Washington, DC: World Bank.

Khan, M. M., F. Sakauchi, T. Sonoda, M. Washio, and M. Mori. 2003. "Magnitude of Arsenic Toxicity in Tube-well Drinking Water in Bangladesh and its Adverse Effects on Human Health Including Cancer: Evidence from a Review of the Literature." *Asian Pacific Journal of Cancer Prevention* 4: 7–14.

Kibriya, M., L. Ali, N. G. Banik, and A. K. A. Khan. 1999. "Home Monitoring of Blood Glucose (HMBG) in Type-2 Diabetes Mellitus in a Developing Country." *Diabetes Research and Clinical Practice* 46 (3): 253–57.

Koehlmoos, T. 2010. "The Hidden Burden of Women Smokers in Bangladesh." BMJ Group Blogs, July 8, 2010. http://blogs.bmj.com/bmj/2010/07/08/tracey-koehlmoos-the-hidden-burden-of-women-smokers-in-bangladesh/.

Koehlmoos, T., Z. Islam, S. Hossain, S. Anwar, R. Gazi, P. K. Streatfield, and A. Bhuiya. 2011. "Health Transcends Poverty: The Bangladesh Experience." In '*Good Health at Low Cost' 25 Years on: What Makes an Effective Health System?*, edited by D. Balabanova, M. McKee, and A. Mills. London: London School of Hygiene & Tropical Medicine.

Koehlmoos, T., M. J. Uddin, A. Ashraf, and M. Rashid. 2009. "Homeless in Dhaka: Violence, Sexual Harassment, and Drug-Abuse." *Journal of Health, Population and Nutrition* 27 (4): 452–61.

Mahmud, I., Z. A. Ahsan, and M. Claeson. 2011. *Drug Use among Street Children and Adolescents in Urban Bangladesh*. Dhaka: World Bank.

Mahtab, H., and M. P. Chowdhury. 2002. "Rural Women: The Bangladesh Perspective." *Diabetes Voice* 47 (Special issue): 34–8.

MIS-DGHS (Management Information System-Directorate General of Health Services). 2009. *Health Bulletin 2008*. Dhaka: Ministry of Health and Family Welfare.

———. 2010. *Health Bulletin 2010*. Dhaka: Ministry of Health and Family Welfare.

MOST (USAID Micronutrient Program). 2004. *Elements of a National Food-Fortification Program for Bangladesh*. Arlington, TX: MOST. http://www.mostproject.org/IVACG/ BangFoodFortPrgm.pdf.

Murray, C. J. L., et al. 2012. "Disability-adjusted Life Years (DALYs) for 291 Diseases and Injuries in 21 Regions, 1990–2010: A Systematic Analysis for the Global Burden of Disease Study 2010." *The Lancet* 380 (9858): 2197–223.

Murray, C. J. L., and A. D. Lopez. 1997. "Alternative Projections of Mortality and Disability by Cause 1990–2020: Global Burden of Disease Study." *The Lancet* 349 (9064): 1498–504.

Ng, N., M. Hakimi, H. Van Minh, S. Juvekar, A. Razzzaque, A. Ashraf, S. M. Ahmed, U. Kanungsukkasem, K. Soonthornthada, and T. Huu Bich. 2009. "Prevalence of Physical Inactivity in Nine Rural INDEPTH Health and Demographic Surveillance Systems in Five Asian Countries." *Global Health Action* (Suppl 1): 44–53.

NIPORT (National Institute of Population Research and Training), MEASURE Evaluation, ICDDR,B, and ACPR (National Institute of Population Research and Training, MEASURE Evaluation, International Centre for Diarrhoeal Disease Research, Bangladesh, and Associates for Community and Population Research). 2008. *2006 Bangladesh Urban Health Survey*. Dhaka: NIPORT, ICDDR,B, ACPR; Chapel Hill, NC: MEASURE Evaluation.

NIPORT, MEASURE Evaluation, and ICDDR,B. 2011. *Bangladesh Maternal Mortality and Health Care Survey 2010: Summary of Key Findings and Implications*. Dhaka: NIPORT, ICDDR,B; Chapel Hill, NC: MEASURE Evaluation.

NIPORT, Mitra and Associates, and ICF International. 2013. *Bangladesh Demographic and Health Survey 2011*. Dhaka.

NIPORT, Mitra and Associates, and Macro International. 2009. *Bangladesh Demographic and Health Survey 2007*. Dhaka: U.S. Agency for International Development, NIPORT, Macro International.

NIPORT, Mitra and Associates, and MEASURE DHS ICF. 2012. *Bangladesh Demographic and Health Survey 2011: Preliminary Report*. Dhaka.

Nonnemaker, J., and M. Sur. 2007. "Tobacco Expenditures and Child Health and Nutritional Outcomes in Rural Bangladesh." *Social Science and Medicine* 65 (12): 2517–26.

Pandey, M. R. 1984. "Domestic Smoke Pollution and Chronic Bronchitis in a Rural Community of the Hill Region of Nepal." *Thorax* 39: 337–39.

Qureshi, K. A. 1994. "Domestic Smoke Pollution and Prevalence of Chronic Bronchitis/ Asthma in a Rural Area of Kashmir." *Indian Journal of Chest Diseases and Allied Sciences* 36 (2): 61–72.

Rahim, M. A. 2008. "Epidemiology of Diabetes in Bangladesh." Unpublished dissertation, Faculty of Medicine, University of Oslo, Oslo.

Rahim, M. A., A. Hussain, A. K. Azad Khan, M. A. Sayeed, S. M. Keramat Ali, and S. Vaaler. 2007. "Rising Prevalence of Type 2 Diabetes in Rural Bangladesh: A Population-based Study." *Diabetes Research and Clinical Practice* 77 (2): 300–05.

Rahim, M. A., A. K. A. Khan, Q. Nahar, S. M. K. Ali, and A. Hussain. 2010. "Impaired Fasting Glucose and Impaired Glucose Tolerance in Rural Population of Bangladesh." *Bangladesh Medical Research Council Bulletin* 36 (2): 47–51.

Ramaraj, R., and P. Chellappa. 2008. "Cardiovascular Risk in South Asians." *Postgraduate Medical Journal* 84 (996): 518–23.

Razzaque, A., L. Nahar, H. V. Minh, N. Ng, S. Juvekar, A. Ashraf, S. M. Ahmed, K. Soonthornthada, U. Kanungsukkasem, and T. Huu Bich. 2009. "Social Factors and Overweight: Evidence from Nine Asian INDEPTH Network Sites." *Global Health Action* 2 (Suppl 1). doi:10.3402/gha.v2i0.1991.

Razzaque, A., L. Nahar, A. H. M. G. Mustafa, Z. A. Karar, M. S. Islam, and M. Yunus. 2011. "Socio-Demographic Differentials of Selected Noncommunicable Diseases Risk Factors among Adults in Matlab, Bangladesh: Findings from a WHO STEPS Survey." *Asia-Pacific Journal of Public Health* 23 (2): 183–91.

Sankaranarayanan, R., N. Bhatla, P. E. Gravitt, P. Basu, P. O. Esmy, K. S. Ashrafunnessa, Y. Ariyaratne, A. Shah, and B. M. Nene. 2008. "Human Papillomavirus Infection and Cervical Cancer Prevention in India, Bangladesh, Sri Lanka and Nepal." *Vaccine* 26 (Supplement 12): M43–52.

Sayeed, M. A., A. Banu, J. A. Haq, P. A. Khanam, H. Mahtab, and A. K. Azad Khan. 2002. "Prevalence of Hypertension in Bangladesh: Effect of Socioeconomic Risk Factor on Difference between Rural and Urban Community." *Bangladesh Medical Research Council Bulletin* 28 (1): 7–18.

Shobhana, R., P. R. Rao, A. Lavanya, V. Vijay, and A. Ramachandran. 2000. "Cost Burden to Diabetic Patients with Foot Complications: A Study from Southern India." *Journal of the Association of Physicians of India* 48 (12): 1147–50.

SIDA (Swedish International Development Cooperation Agency). 2009. *Reality Check Bangladesh 2008: Listening to the Poor People's Realities about Primary Healthcare and Primary Education*. Dhaka: Edita Communications.

Siddique, M. A., M. A. U. Sultan, K. M. H. S. S. Haque, M. M. Zaman, C. M. Ahmed, M. A. Rahim, and M. Salman. 2008. "Clustering of Metabolic Factors among the Patients with Essential Hypertension." *Bangladesh Medical Research Council Bulletin* 34 (3): 71–5.

Smith, G. D. 2007. "Life-Course Approaches to Inequalities in Adult Chronic Disease Risk." *Proceedings of the Nutrition Society* 66 (2): 216–36.

Smith, A. H., C. Hopenhayn-Rich, M. N. Bates, H. M. Goeden, I. Hertz-Picciotto, H. M. Duggan, R. Wood, M. J. Kosnett, and M. T. Smith. 1992. "Cancer Risks from Arsenic in Drinking Water." *Environmental Health Perspectives* 97: 259–67.

Smith, A. H., E. O. Lingas, and M. Rahman. 2000. "Contamination of Drinking-Water by Arsenic in Bangladesh: A Public Health Emergency." *Bulletin of the World Health Organization* 78 (9): 1093–103.

Talukdar, S. I., M. A. Haque, M. O. Alam, M. H. Huq, M. S. Ali, C. R. Debnath, M. M. Rashid, A. Roushan, M. K. Jahan, K. Nahar, and A. Khanom. 2007. "Histopathology-Based Cancer Pattern in Mymensingh Region of Bangladesh." *Mymensingh Medical Journal* 16 (2): 165–9.

UNICEF (United Nations Children's Fund). 2008. "Arsenic Mitigation in Bangladesh." http://www.unicef.org/bangladesh/Arsenic.pdf.

UNICEF and BBS (Bangladesh Bureau of Statistics). 2005. *National Low Birth Weight Survey of Bangladesh: 2003–2004*. Dhaka: BBS with assistance from UNICEF.

UNICEF and WHO (World Health Organization). 2004. *Low Birthweight: Country, Regional and Global Estimates*. New York: UNICEF.

Wang, H., N. M. Shara, D. Calhoun, J. G. Umans, E. T. Lee, and B. V. Howard. 2010. "Incidence Rates and Predictors of Diabetes in Those with Prediabetes: The Strong Heart Study." *Diabetes-Metabolism Research and Reviews* 26 (5): 378–85. doi:10.1002/dmrr.1089.

Watts, C., and A. Cairncross. 2012. "Should the GBD Risk Factor Ranking be Used to Guide Policy?" Comment on GBD 2010. *The Lancet* 380: 2060–61.

WHO (World Health Organization). 2003. *World Health Report 2003: Today's Challenges.* Geneva, Switzerland.

———. 2004. *Global Status Report on Alcohol 2004.* http://apapaonline.org/data/National_Data/Bangladesh/Situation_Bangladesh.pdf.

———. 2005. *Preventing Chronic Diseases: A Vital Investment.* WHO Global Report, Geneva, Switzerland. http://www.who.int/chp/chronic_disease_report/contents/en/index.html.

———. 2006. "World Mortality Country Factsheet 2006: Bangladesh." Geneva

———. 2007. *Indoor Air Pollution: National Burden of Disease Estimates.* Geneva.

———. 2008a. "Disease and Injury Regional Estimates: Cause-Specific Mortality: Regional Estimates for 2008." http://www.who.int/healthinfo/global_burden_disease/estimates_regional/en/index.html.

———. 2008b. *WHO Report on the Global Tobacco Epidemic, 2008: The MPOWER Package.* Geneva.

———. 2009a. *World Health Statistics 2009.* Geneva.

———. 2009b. "Bangladesh." In *Global Status Report on Road Safety.* Geneva. http://www.who.int/violence_injury_prevention/road_safety_status/report/country_profiles_all_en.pdf.

———. 2010. *Creating an Enabling Environment for Population-based Salt Reduction Strategies.* Geneva, Switzerland: WHO; London: Food Standards Agency. http://whqlibdoc.who.int/publications/2010/9789241500777_eng.pdf.

———. 2011a. *WHO Report on the Global Tobacco Epidemic, 2011. Warning about the Dangers of Tobacco.* Geneva.

———. 2011b. *Global Status Report on Alcohol and Health 2011.* Geneva.

WHO BD (World Health Organization, Country Office for Bangladesh). 2009. *Global Adult Tobacco Survey: Bangladesh Country Report 2009.* Dhaka. http://www.who.int/tobacco/surveillance/global_adult_tobacco_survey_bangladesh_report_2009.pdf.

———. 2011. *Bangladesh NCD Risk Factor Survey 2010.* Dhaka.

WHO SEARO (World Health Organization, Regional Office for South East Asia). 2007a. *Impact of Tobacco-Related Illnesses in Bangladesh,* edited by M. M. Zaman, N. Nargis, A. Perucic, and K. Rahman. New Delhi: WHO SEARO. http://www.ban.searo.who.int/LinkFiles/Publication_Tobacco_Free_Initiative_Health_Cost_ban.pdf.

————. 2007b. "Scaling Up Preventions and Control of Chronic Non-Communicable Diseases in the SEA Region: Risk Factors for Non-Communicable Diseases (Results from Surveys Using the WHO STEPS Approach)." Regional Committee Document, New Delhi.

World Bank. 2006. "Bangladesh Country Environmental Analysis." Bangladesh Development Series Paper 12, Dhaka.

————. 2008. *Sri Lanka: Addressing the Needs of an Aging Population.* Report 43396-LK. Human Development Unit, South Asia Region. Washington, DC. http://siteresources .worldbank.org/INTSRILANKA/Resources/LKAgingFullRep.pdf.

Zaman, M. M., and M. A. Rouf. 1999. "Prevalence of Hypertension in a Bangladeshi Adult Population." *Journal of Human Hypertension* 13: 547–49.

CHAPTER 3

Health System and NCD Capacity Assessment

Introduction

The prevention and management of noncommunicable diseases (NCDs) are largely governed by the capacity of the health system, yet capacity assessments of the system can be more challenging than burden of disease (BOD) assessments and tend to be conducted less frequently.

The World Health Organization (WHO) models the health system with six building blocks that contribute to strengthening health systems in different ways (figure 3.1). Some cross-cutting components, such as *leadership/governance* and *information*, provide the basis for the overall policy and regulation of all the other health system blocks. Key input components include *financing* and the *health workforce*. A third group, namely *medical products and technologies* and *service delivery*, reflects the immediate outputs of the health system, that is, the availability and distribution of care (WHO 2007). An analysis of each of these building blocks provides an assessment of the overall system's capacity to manage NCDs (see box 3.1).

Health Service Delivery

Government Structure

An original signatory of the Alma Ata Declaration in 1978, Bangladesh developed a government health system along the Health for All model. According to the Constitution, ensuring provision of medical care, raising the level of nutritional status, and improving public health of all citizens are the primary responsibilities of the state.

The National Health Policy 2001 is being updated in line with the National Development Strategy and National Poverty Reduction Plan to ensure that access to health services is pro-poor. The new health policy promises to continue focusing on existing and emerging diseases and threats to the health status of the population. It also shows increased commitment to health sector reform by

Box 3.1 Chapter Three Summary

The assessment of the health system's capacity to manage NCDs is considered under the following headings:

- Health Service Delivery. The government's role in NCDs is limited to providing health education at primary level and preventive and clinical treatment at tertiary level, with less focus on preventive clinical care at primary and secondary levels, while the private sector provides mainly treatment services. NGOs, private providers (formal and informal), and traditional medicine play a large role in service delivery. The National Health Policy 2001 is being updated to ensure that access to health services is pro-poor. A few strategies and guidelines on NCDs exist but there is no good awareness-raising system to keep policy makers abreast of these concerns.
- Health Workforce. In 2007 the country had an estimated 7.7 qualified health care providers per 10,000 of the population (WHO recommends 25). Physicians and nurses account for only 5 percent of health care providers. Most health care providers are informally trained and cater to the needs of the majority, particularly the poor. Until recently, few health workers are trained in NCD prevention and management, but in 2013 the number has been increasing.
- Health Information Systems. Bangladesh has no community public health program or national surveillance for NCDs. Only specialized, tertiary-level hospital-based information is available. Some NCD risk factors are being addressed in Dhaka's population by the National Institute of Preventive and Social Medicine (NIPSOM) and BIRDEM.
- Pharmaceuticals. The pharmaceutical sector is thriving with a national essential drugs policy, and drugs for treating NCDs were only recently included in the list of essential drugs.
- Health Financing. Total health expenditure (public and private) accounted for 3.5 percent of GDP in 2011. Per capita health expenditure—inadequate to secure basic services—was about $23 in 2011, a third government financed. Although the budget allocated for the NCD line directorate increased to $70 million for 2011–2016, this and the portion allocated for NCD awareness are not enough to address the growing NCDs challenges, particularly CVDs.
- Health Sector Governance. Overall government effectiveness is weak, having deteriorated significantly since 2000. Accountability and regulatory quality are also low. Tackling NCDs requires an effective governance system to coordinate the multisectoral interventions, a strong regulatory framework to issue new laws and regulations, and increased capacity to enforce them.

strengthening the government's stewardship role to deliver health services and its regulatory capacity among the whole sector.

In line with the general system of public administration in Bangladesh, the Ministry of Health and Family Welfare (MOHFW) management structure comprises two main groupings, both headed by the secretary under the leadership of the minister (figure 3.2):

- The secretariat, responsible for policy development and administration, comprising eight functional wings and units headed by a joint secretary or a joint chief; and

Figure 3.1 Building Blocks of a Health System

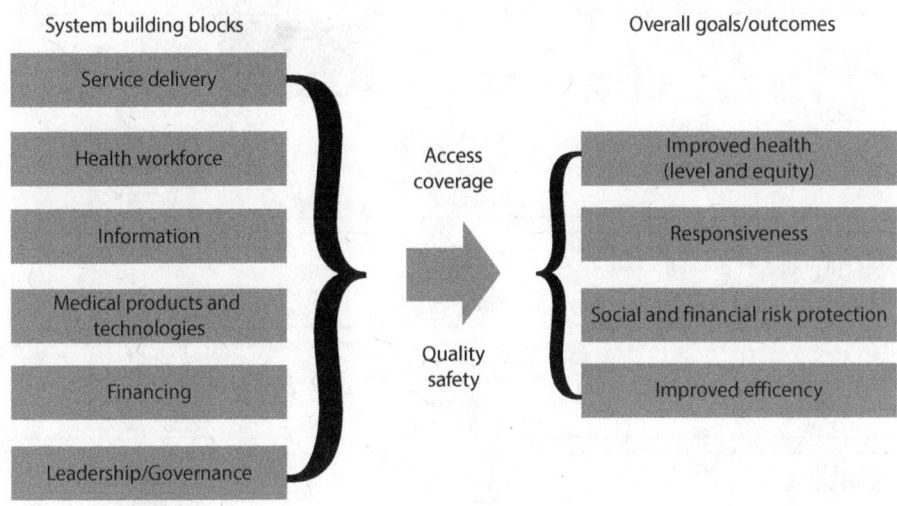

Source: WHO 2007.

- Executing agencies, through which the MOHFW implements its programs and policies, comprising 10 directorates, units, and institutions.

The executing agencies include the Directorate General of Health Services (DGHS) and the Directorate General of Family Planning (DGFP), each led by a director general (DG) supported by additional DGs, line directors, and hospital or specialist agency directors. Both directorates have separate management and delivery structures from national to union/ward level. Since 2003, there has been a line director for Public Health Intervention and Non-Communicable Disease Control who serves within the DGHS (see chapter 4). Under the NCD line director are the programs for Non-Communicable Diseases/Health of Senior Citizens, Adolescents and Disabled; Arsenic; and Occupational and Environmental Health.

At present, there are two program managers working under the line director, including a newly created position for managing the NCD program. Until recently, the emphasis within the NCD line directorate was on arsenic and less on major NCDs and injuries.

The mandate for providing primary health care in urban areas is with the Ministry of Local Government, Rural Development and Co-operatives. Primary health care services provided directly by the DGHS are, therefore, confined to those supplied by medical college hospital outpatient departments, district hospitals, government outpatient dispensaries, and maternal and child health services provided by the Family Planning Directorate. Urban primary health care, apart from for-profit private providers, is mainly provided in all the six city corporations and five selected municipalities of Bangladesh by nongovermental organizations (NGOs) under the Urban Primary Health Care Project (UPHCP) financed by the government, Asian Development Bank, Department for

Figure 3.2 Structure of the Health Service Delivery System in the MOHFW

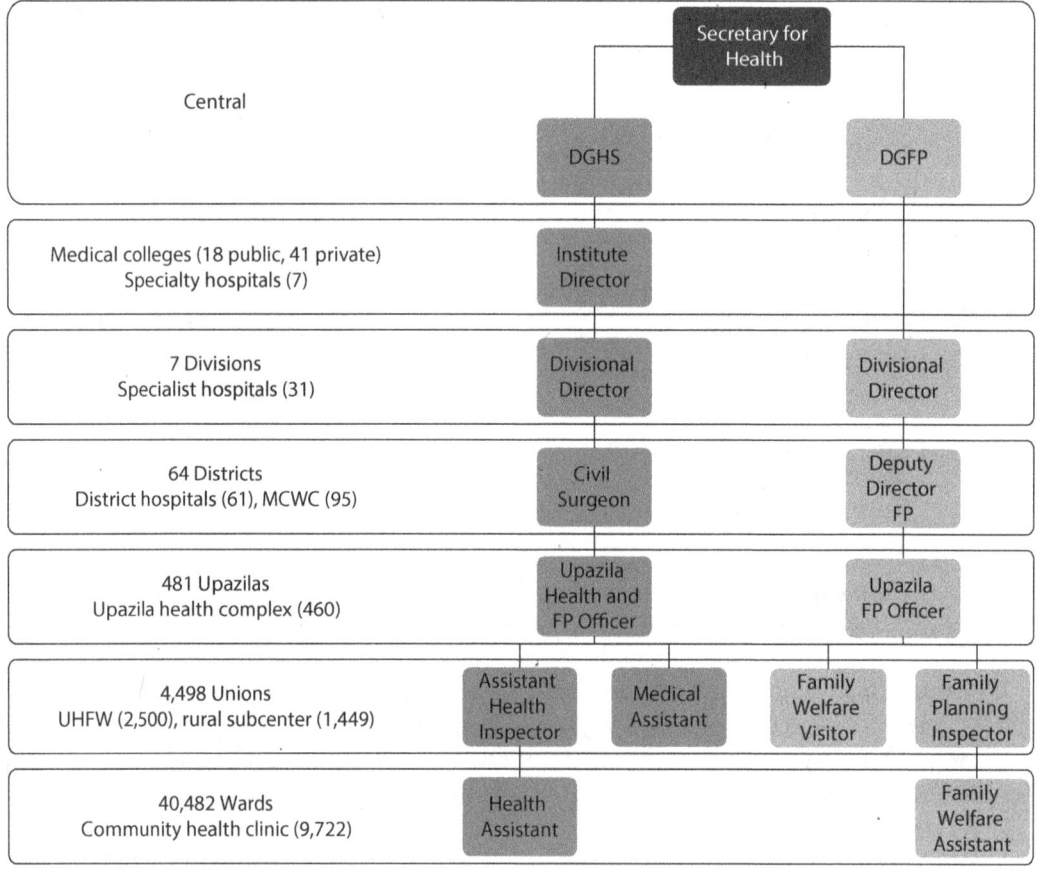

Source: MIS-DGHS 2010.
Note: DGHS = Directorate General of Health Services; DGFP = Directorate General of Family Planning; MOHFW = Ministry of Health and Family
Welfare. MCWC = Maternal and Child Welfare Center; UHFWC = Union Health and Family Welfare Center

International Development (DFID) of the United Kingdom, Swedish International Development Cooperation Agency (SIDA), United Nations Population Fund (UNFPA), and ORBIS International. NCDs are not a priority for the UPHCP (UPHCP 2010).

Nonpublic Sector

The nonpublic sector also plays a significant role, via three main groups: NGOs; private providers (formal and informal); and traditional medicine. The largest NGO in the world, Bangladesh Rural Advancement Committee (BRAC), is based in Bangladesh and touches the lives of more than 110 million Bangladeshi citizens with its 64,000 village health workers, who, as well as providing basic health services, work with the government to deliver Directly Observed Treatment—Short course (DOTS) to tuberculosis (TB) patients in rural areas. Discussions are under way between BRAC and the Diabetic Association of

Bangladesh to incorporate elements of diabetes management and prevention into the package of services delivered at the community level by the *Shasthya Shebika* (community health workers).

Other large NGOs work primarily with rural or disadvantaged populations. Innovations such as a large social franchising organization work within the NGO sector. Funded by the United States Agency for International Development (USAID), the Smiling Sun Franchising Program is the first such program to have a primary health care focus rather than delivering services for a vertical program. It intends to include NCD management in its service package (details are under discussion).

The private sector is large and complex. The formal sector has multiple hospitals and clinics in urban areas and municipalities, but dual practice, licensing, and absenteeism between public and private sector providers are pervasive issues. There is a general belief that most chronic illnesses and acute incidents are treated in the private sector (Engelgau *et al.* 2011; SIDA 2009), but there is no reporting between the nonstate and public sectors (HLSP/Mott McDonald Ltd. 2010). The for-profit modern health care sector is mostly in urban areas, particularly the larger cities. Over the last decade, these services have been extending to some flourishing *upazilas*.

During 1982–2010, the DGHS registered 2,501 private hospitals and clinics. Total bed capacity of this sector is about 52 percent of the national total (MIS-DGHS 2010). About 5,122 diagnostic centers had registered with the MOHFW through 2010, with increasing investments in state-of-the-art diagnostic tests and services. Private diagnostic centers now account for the largest share of this sector, but their proliferation may not be justified; also, their quality is frequently called into question. The Bangladesh National Health Accounts 1997–2007 estimates that expenditure in private/NGO hospitals in 2007 was about $34.0 million, or 54.0 percent of total outlays on hospital services. This estimate is nearly double the 1997 share (22.5 percent of total expenditure on hospitals, or $28.3 million).

In 2003, 43 percent of service users visited unqualified practitioners for curative care, and another 13 percent obtained treatment from drug shops (Cockroft, Milne, and Andersson 2004). The traditional medicine systems practiced in Bangladesh include *Unani* and *Ayurvedic*, which have a joint governing board, although each has its own network of teaching colleges. The expansive informal sector includes traditional birth attendants, drug vendors, and village doctors. While reliable figures on the numbers of these different types of informal practitioners are lacking, the Bangladesh Health Labor Market Study has estimated the total number of private practitioners in Bangladesh to be around 0.45 million, or 3.6 per 1,000 population in 2003. Of these, traditional and unqualified providers outnumber formally qualified ones by 12 to 1 (Peters and Kayne 2003). More recent estimates indicate that 94 percent of the health workforce in Bangladesh is composed of unqualified health care providers, including traditional healers, village doctors, and drug sellers (BHW 2008). Private health expenditure is growing faster than public expenditure, and for-profit providers responded by expanding their range of services and by increasing their share in total health expenditure by about 15 percent annually in 2001–07 (HEU 2010).

Bangladesh has a very high volume of use of private practitioners for first-line curative care, including among the poor. Because public sector infrastructure at primary care level in rural areas offers an Essential Services Package that has no components addressing NCDs and no paramedics trained in management of NCDs, users seeking treatment for these conditions are thought to go very largely to the private formal and informal sectors, including pharmacies (licensed or unlicensed). The same situation prevails in urban areas where the UPHCP deliver the same Essential Services Package as in rural areas. Rural areas have limited numbers of physicians, and people routinely turn to the unlicensed providers and traditional healers for treatment—NCDs are no exception. Diabetes, stroke, heart disease, and their symptoms are usually treated outside the formal health care system by unlicensed providers (Bhuiya 2009).

Specialized Institutes

The National Institute of Cardiovascular Diseases (NICVD) is the apex specialized public hospital that provides clinical care services to prevent and treat chronic cardiovascular diseases (CVDs). The National Centre for Control of Rheumatic Fever and Heart Diseases (NCCRFHD) provides clinical care for rheumatic heart diseases. The National Institute of Cancer Research and Hospital (NICRH) is the national focal point and referral center for cancer treatment. The National Institute of Mental Health and Research (NIMHR), Pabna Mental Hospital, National Asthma Centre, and the National Institute of Kidney Diseases and Urology (NIKDU) are other specialized institutes that provide clinical care for different NCDs.

Understandably, the patient loads for specialized public institutes are enormous—in 2009, NICVD alone catered to 41,555 and 160,008 people in its in- and outpatient departments, respectively. Bangladesh Institute of Research and Rehabilitation in Diabetes, Endocrine and Metabolic Disorders (BIRDEM) and National Heart Foundation Hospital and Research Institute (NHFH&RI) are the leading nongovernment service providers for diabetes and heart disease, respectively (MIS-DGHS 2010).

Beyond these public and NGO institutes are tertiary private hospitals, which provide emergency and curative care for CVD and other NCDs. The Centre for the Rehabilitation of the Paralysed is the leading private organization providing clinical care for spinal injury and disabilities. The Centre for Injury Prevention and Research, Bangladesh, is engaged in advocacy, research, and training to prevent accidents and injuries.

Currently, NCDs are tackled at the secondary and tertiary levels that mostly provide treatment in specialized facilities; there is less emphasis on prevention at the primary care level and using readily available low-cost treatment interventions. Much of the investment in the infrastructure and medical equipment in the specialized hospitals may be saved if NCDs prevention interventions are scaled up.

Challenges

The government's health service delivery for NCDs is limited to providing health education at primary level and preventive and clinical treatment at tertiary level, with less focus on preventive clinical care at primary and secondary levels. The Upazila NCD Project (launched in 2007) and the NCD Control and Public Health Intervention program have provided training to public and private providers to develop NCD capacity and increase awareness of NCDs among senior citizens (Bleich et al. 2010) but its scope remains limited. Also, a few strategies and guidelines on NCDs exist but there is no good awareness-raising system to keep policy makers abreast of these concerns.

In addressing the Millennium Development Goal (MDG) challenges, the health service delivery system in Bangladesh, similar to that in most developing countries, was structured to deal with "episodes" of maternal and child health illnesses and communicable diseases. The shifting in the BOD toward NCDs would require adopting an integrated approach that ensures continuity care. A capacity assessment conducted by WHO in all the 11 Member States of the South-East Asia Region in 2006–07 indicated that, except for a very high commitment to tobacco control, Bangladesh health service delivery has limited capacity with regard to prevention and control of NCDs (WHO SEARO 2007).

Health Workforce

Recent MOHFW staff positions include 39,327 physicians, 2,299 dentists, and 23,056 nurses in the public sector along with 5,746 family welfare visitors; 5,598 medical assistants; and 12,441 medical technologists (HLSP/Mott MacDonald Ltd. 2010). Other government health facilities exist for specific groups (for example, the police, defense, and Bangladesh Railways), and the MOHFW does not play a role in managing these facilities, though the number of their physicians and nurses is less than 200 (Hossain and Hussain 2009). The Ministry of Local Government, Rural Development and Co-operatives is responsible for the delivery of health services to the urban population. The 2007 estimate of total health workforce density is 146 per 10,000 population, with a ratio of 7.7 per 10,000 qualified health care providers (BHW 2008) compared with a WHO-recommended 25.0 per 10,000 population (WHO 2006a). Figure 3.3 illustrates the different types of health care providers in Bangladesh.

Others includes circumcision practitioners, tooth extractors, ear cleaners, and so on.

The largest group of health care providers is the informally trained (including village doctors, drug sellers, kobiraj, totka, herbalists, faith healers, and untrained traditional birth attendants), who cater to the needs of the majority of the population, particularly the poor, with traditional healers and traditional birth attendants (trained and untrained) accounting for 44 and 22 percent of all health care providers.

Physicians and nurses represent only 5 percent of health care providers—with about five physicians and two nurses per 10,000 population. However, there are

Figure 3.3 Types of Health Care Providers in Bangladesh, 2007

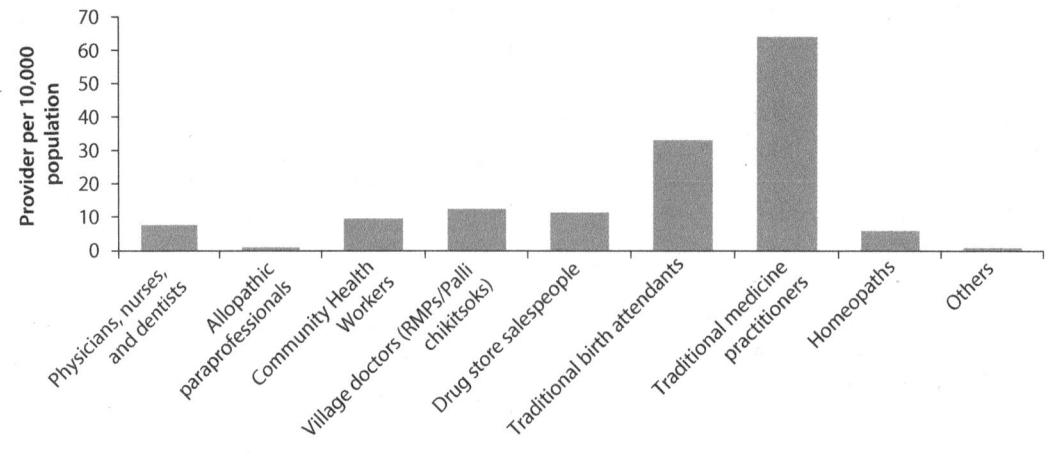

Source: BHW 2008.

substantial variations in the density of physicians and nurses among the divisions (most are in Dhaka, followed by Chittagong) as well as an urban–rural difference, with the majority of qualified providers in urban areas. Lack of incentives for recruitment and retention of health workers in rural areas has led to staff shortages, and absenteeism rates are high, as providers work part time privately. With greater proliferation of technologies in health care, the requirement of human resources in health in appropriate numbers, skill mix, and at the right place (to deliver the Essential Services Package, including NCD prevention and treatment) will remain a challenge.

Few health workers are trained in NCD prevention and management (WHO BD 2010), but in 2013 the number has been increasing. The apex training institutes in the public sector are National Institute of Preventive and Social Medicine (NIPSOM) for public health training; NICVD, which offers postgraduate courses on cardiology and training of nurses and paramedics for CVD; and the National Institute of Diseases of Chest & Hospital, which offers postgraduate training on chest diseases (medical and surgical).

In the nongovernment sector, BIRDEM opened the Bangladesh Institute for Health Sciences Academy to produce qualified human resources for all medical institutions in the country. NHFH&RI has postgraduate courses for physicians (MD cardiology and MS cardiothoracic surgery), nurses (advanced cardiac nursing), and technologists (such as perfusion technologists and cath-lab technicians). However, the total postgraduate medical training capacity from all government and private institutions is only 2,222 a year, and the specialized public and private NCD institutes constitute only 11 percent of total capacity.

The Bangladesh College of Physicians and Surgeons offers various fellowships and memberships on specific subject areas, but during 2006–09, no fellowship was provided in cardiology. (The total number of fellowships/memberships in

NCDs such as cardiology, psychiatry, and thoracic surgery were 22 out of 1,164 during the period.) Despite Bangladesh managing a nationwide network of 59 medical colleges (41 of them private), 13 nursing colleges (7 private), 69 nursing institutes (22 private), 17 medical assistant training schools (10 private), and 16 institutes of health technology (13 private) (MIS-DGHS 2010), WHO identified Bangladesh as among 57 countries with a critical shortage of doctors, nurses, and midwives (WHO 2006b).

Health Information Systems

Health information systems data are collected by the public health facilities at district level and below. Tertiary and nonstate sector providers and facilities are generally in poor compliance with requests for reporting (MIS-DGHS 2009). This information includes disease-specific morbidity and mortality based on 37 selected diseases, including NCDs. Reports are filed monthly. To increase data collection, plans are under way to make the paper reporting systems into an electronic reporting system, and to that effect, there are plans to equip each *upazila* with a wireless modem and to test the outfitting of village health workers with handheld devices (MIS-DGHS 2009).

The Management Information System (MIS) of the DGHS collects information from 6 postgraduate institute hospitals, 6 medical college hospitals, and 64 districts (including district and other hospitals and all the public health facilities below them). Statistical staff in the hospitals code mortality events into the International Statistical Classification of Diseases (ICD-10). Forty major conditions are used to classify deaths. The information gathered by the MIS is shared with the nation through the annual *Health Bulletin*. The DGHS and MIS maintain websites that feature activities and some statistical information. The Institute of Epidemiology, Disease Control and Research (IEDCR) has been implementing the Behavioral Risk Factor Surveillance System, Bangladesh, on a pilot basis to collect information on health conditions and risk behaviors contributing to NCDs, injuries, and preventable communicable diseases. This is a computerized mobile phone–based surveillance system, which was established with technical support from Centers for Disease Control and Prevention, Atlanta, Georgia, and financial assistance from the International Association of National Public Health Institutes.

Because most care is sought in the nonstate sector, there are limits to what the MIS captures. For this reason, the DGHS has conducted "geographic reconnaissance" each year in January–February at the household level, recording births, deaths, and other changes in family information for about 30 million families. The last reconnaissance report was published in 2004 using data collected in 2002. Building on the national identification project of 2007–08 and the National Census of 2011, changes are being made to expand the scope of data collection (which may cover NCDs) and extend the period to six months (MIS-DGHS 2009).

Bangladesh has no community public health program or national surveillance for NCDs, and only hospital-based information from specialized tertiary-level hospitals is available. Recently, the Cancer Institute has taken the initiative for a cancer registry, and the NCCRFHD has started registration of rheumatic heart disease cases in Dhaka and outlying rural health complexes. Some NCD risk factors are being addressed in the population of Dhaka by NIPSOM and BIRDEM, and coverage is being expanded to other divisions (WHO BD 2010).

Pharmaceuticals and Medical Technology

The pharmaceutical sector in Bangladesh is thriving, with about 224 licensed pharmaceutical factories, 6 of which are owned by multinational companies that account for about 10.4 percent of local production. Around 85.0 percent of the raw materials used in local production of pharmaceuticals are imported and only 1.1 percent of locally produced drugs are exported. In a speech to Parliament on 11 June 2009, the Minister of Finance recommended developing the pharmaceutical sector for exports.

The Directorate of Drugs Administration, under the MOHFW, has responsibility for administering, controlling, and managing the pharmaceutical sector. The directorate is the regulatory agency implementing drug laws and monitoring the quality of finished products. At present, about 450 generic drugs, in 5,300 registered brands having 8,300 different presentations of dosage forms and strengths, are manufactured in the pharmaceutical sector. However, the local market is extremely concentrated, with the top 10 firms capturing about 70 percent. Two companies alone, Beximco and Square, hold 25 percent of the market.

Since the 1980s, Bangladesh has had a national essential drugs policy and an essential drugs list to be procured and used in public health services. Most of the essential drugs are generics. Production and distribution facilities exist primarily in the public sector and with few private companies. Major innovation during the mid-1990s helped to alleviate the previous gap between supply and demand for essential drugs in public health facilities. Drugs for treating NCDs were included recently in the essential drugs list (with technical assistance from WHO).

As for medical equipment, out of the total five-year budget of $65.0 million for the NCD operational plan, about $2.5 million is allocated for equipment such as blood pressure machines, lipid profile kits, diabitometers, and nebulizers. In the meantime, the operational plan of the Improved Hospital Service Management had an allocation of about $17 million for high-end equipment for NCDs (for the first 18 months only), which, if extrapolated to the five-year plan, would come to about $60 million.[1] More emphasis on prevention and early detection would require shifting more resources to the primary care level, which would eventually reduce the investments needed in high-end equipment.

Health Financing

In 2011, total expenditure on health accounted for 3.5 percent of gross domestic product (GDP) in Bangladesh, and per capita health expenditure was about $23, of which a third was financed by the government ($7.80). Although total

Figure 3.4 Share of Public Health Expenditure in Total Health Expenditure and in Total Public Expenditure

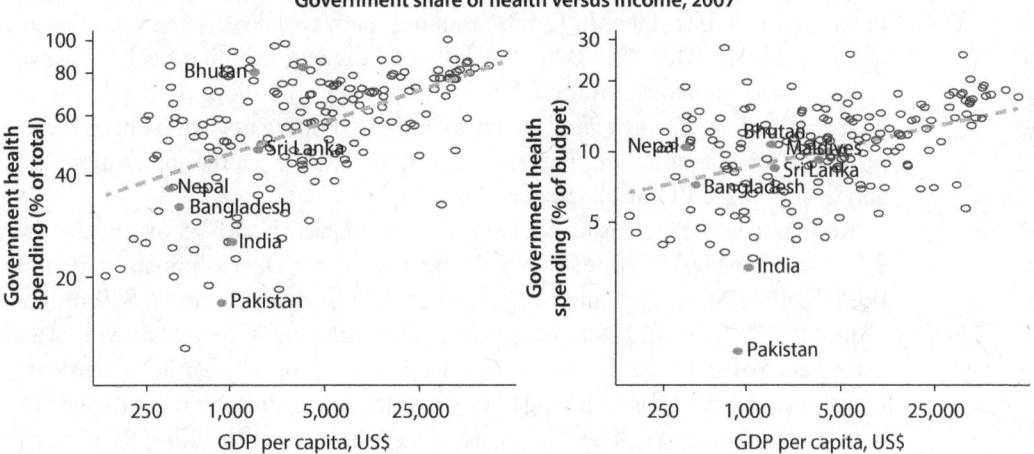

Government share of health versus income, 2007

Source: World Development Indicators, WHO, and Royal Monetary Authority, 2009. Health expenditure data are preliminary as of May 2009; Gottret and Schieber 2010.
Note: Log scale. GDP = gross domestic product.

expenditure on health as a share of GDP had declined during 2000–07, there was an increase in general government spending on health as a share of total expenditure on health in the same period (31.8 percent in 2007 versus 26.5 percent in 2000) (WHO 2009). Compared with other countries of comparable incomes, the Government of Bangladesh spent less on health as a share of total public expenditure (figure 3.4).

Nearly 86 percent of private expenditure is out of pocket. Although services should be no-cost at the point of service in all government facilities, research shows that at least one-quarter of users make extra payments. There is limited utilization and overall poor perceptions of quality in the public sector. Initiatives to increase uptake of services, particularly in MDG priority areas, include a large pilot of a demand-side financing voucher scheme for safe motherhood and a conditional cash transfer for skilled birth attendance at delivery (which stood at 13 percent in 2004).

Household out-of-pocket expenditure at drug outlets accounts for 46 percent of total health expenditure, making household over-the-counter purchases of drugs by far the single largest expenditure item within the sector. In terms of expenditure on the Essential Services Package of the MOHFW (which has six components—child health services, reproductive health care, family planning, limited curative health care, control of communicable diseases, and a program for behavioral change), in 2000/01, 41 percent went to reproductive health including family planning, 40 percent to child health, 14 percent to limited curative care, and 4 percent and 1 percent, respectively, to communicable disease control and behavior change communication (Naripokkho 2006). These figures have likely remained largely unchanged over the last few years.

The NCD line directorate in fiscal year 2008/09 had a total budget of about $10.2 million. The majority of these funds were dedicated to supporting the Institute of Public Health ($4.31 million) and to the program on arsenic ($4.24 million), while $25,000 went to strengthening the NCD cell. However, in the estimated allocation for 2008–11, no money was allotted for piloting the NCD project in the *upazilas*, which included components on training service providers for strengthening prevention services, and for increasing awareness of and diagnosing CVD at *upazila* facilities.

Recognizing the increasing NCD burden, in the new health sector program for 2011–16—the Health, Population and Nutrition Sector Development Programme (HPNSDP)—the budget allocated for the NCD line directorate is $70 million. Out of this, 34 percent is for awareness building, training of service providers, and surveillance of major NCDs including arsenicosis, followed by similar activities for nonconventional NCDs including injury and violence against women (16 percent); emergency preparedness and response and post-disaster health (16 percent); occupational health and safety health issues (11 percent); climate change and other environmental health issues (11 percent); and mental health, tobacco, and substance abuse (11 percent) (Government of Bangladesh 2011).

While the increase in the budget allocated to NCDs reflects a positive trend, the total amount and the portion for NCD awareness are not enough to address growing NCDs challenges, particularly CVDs.

Health Sector Governance

Governance refers to the wide range of functions carried out by governments as they seek to achieve national health policy objectives. Governance is a political process that involves balancing competing influences and demands. It includes maintaining the strategic direction of policy development and implementation; detecting and correcting undesirable trends and distortions; articulating the case for health in national development; regulating the behavior of a wide range of actors, from health care financiers to health care providers; and establishing effective accountability mechanisms (WHO 2010).

Measuring governance is a challenge, however. Kaufman, Kraay, and Mastruzzi (2010) developed an index from several indicators collected by multiple institutions, which assessed six dimensions of governance: voice and accountability; political stability and lack of violence; government effectiveness; regulatory quality; rule of law; and control of corruption—all of which affect the environment for health care services. Figure 3.5 depicts the governance indicators in 2000–09 for Bangladesh. While all these dimensions are important, three are more critical for the health sector—government effectiveness, voice and accountability, and regulatory quality. Yet government effectiveness is low, ranking at around the 18th percentile in 2009, and has shown significant deterioration since 2000. Voice and accountability is also low and did not improve much during the same period. Similarly, regulatory quality has been very low with a ranking in the 24th percentile.

Figure 3.5 Bangladesh Governance Indicators, 2000–09

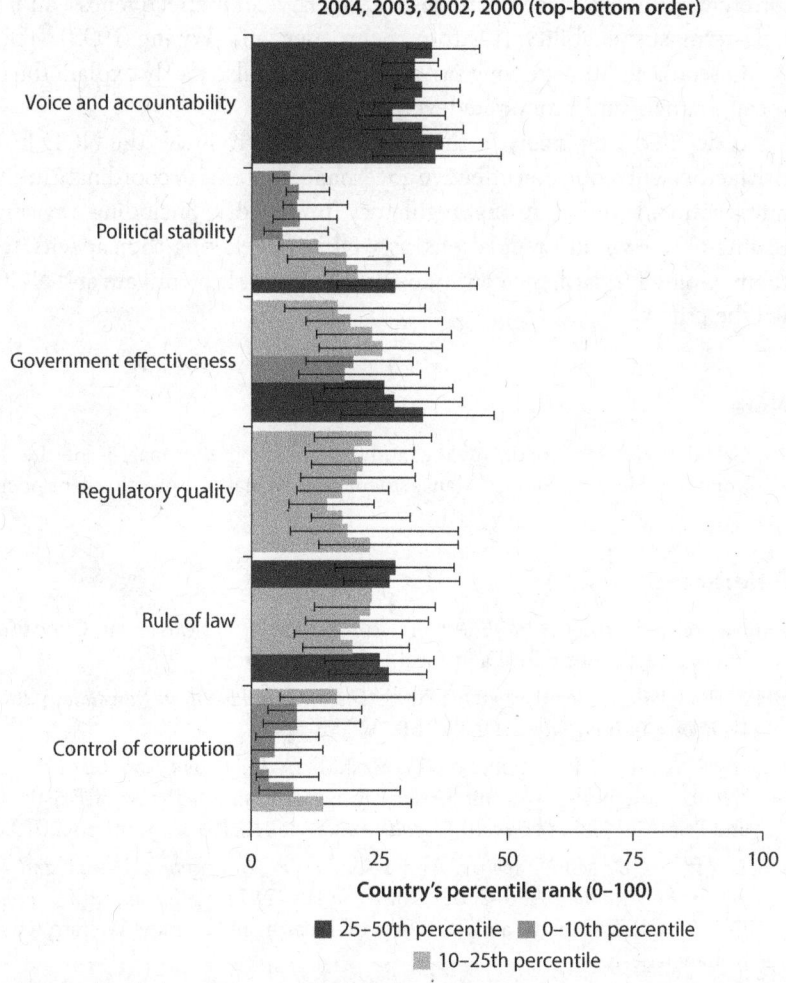

Comparison between 2009, 2008, 2007, 2006, 2005, 2004, 2003, 2002, 2000 (top-bottom order)

Voice and accountability

Political stability

Government effectiveness

Regulatory quality

Rule of law

Control of corruption

Country's percentile rank (0–100)

■ 25–50th percentile   ■ 0–10th percentile
■ 10–25th percentile

Source: Kaufmann, Kraay, and Mastruzzi 2010.
Note: The governance indicators presented here aggregate the views on the quality of governance provided by a large number of enterprise, citizen, and expert survey respondents in industrial and developing countries. These data are gathered from a number of survey institutes, think tanks, nongovernmental organizations, and international organizations. The Worldwide Governance Indicators (WGI) do not reflect the official views of the World Bank, its Executive Directors, or the countries they represent. The WGI are not used by the World Bank Group to allocate resources.

Despite these low governance indicators, Bangladesh has achieved significant progress in poverty reduction, human development, and economic growth, which may be explained by the notion of "polycentric governance." This connotes many centers of decision making that are formally independent of each other but take each other into account in competitive relationships and enter into various contractual and cooperative undertakings that may function in a coherent manner with consistent and predictable patterns of interacting behavior (Ostrom,

Tiebout, and Warren 1961, 831). A system of asymmetric, multi-centric, and overlapping jurisdictions that tackle the economic and technical aspects of different public services can raise efficiency and effectiveness and promote long-term sustainability (Ostrom, Schroeder, and Wynne 1993). The vibrant NGO sector and the growing private sector may also partly explain the country's social, human, and economic development.

As detailed later, many of the policies needed to lower the NCD burden and risk factors will require an effective governance system (to coordinate multisectoral interventions) and a strong regulatory framework, including revising and/or issuing new laws and regulations, as well as developing the capacity to enforce them. Going forward, the continued engagement of the private and NGO sectors will be critical.

Note

1. Calculations were made by the authors based on the analysis of the NCD and Improved Hospital Service Management operational and procurement plans.

References

Bhuiya, A., ed. 2009. *Health for the Rural Masses: Insights from Chakaria*. Dhaka: International Centre for Diarrhoeal Disease Research.

BHW (Bangladesh Health Watch). 2008. *The State of Health in Bangladesh 2007: Health Workforce in Bangladesh*. Dhaka: BRAC University.

Bleich, S. N., T. L. P. Koehlmoos, M. Rashid, D. H. Peters, and G. Anderson. 2010. "Noncommunicable Chronic Disease in Bangladesh: Overview of Existing Programs and Priorities Going Forward." *Health Policy*. doi:10.1016/j.healthpol.2010.09.004.

Cockcroft, A., D. Milne, and N. Andersson. 2004. *Bangladesh Health and Population Sector Programme 1998–2003: Third Service Delivery Survey 2003 Final Report*. Dhaka: CIET Canada and Ministry of Health and Family Welfare, Government of Bangladesh.

Engelgau, M., S. Rosenhouse, S. El-Saharty, and A. Mahal. 2011. "The Economic Effect of Noncommunicable Diseases on Households: A Review of Existing Evidence." *Journal of Health Communications*, 16 (Supplement 2): 75–81.

Gottret, P., and G. Schieber. 2010. Health System Objective & Socioeconomic Overview: Achievements & Challenges; presented in South Asia Regional Forum on Health Financing; Maldives, June 2-4, 2010. http://siteresources.worldbank.org/ HEALTHNUTRITIONANDPOPULATION/Resources/281627-1114107818507/1011070-1281041448823/PabloGottretSAProgressChallenges.pdf

Government of Bangladesh. 2011. *Health Population and Nutrition Sector Development Program 2011–16: Program Implementation Plan*. Vol. 1. Dhaka: Ministry of Health and Family Welfare.

HEU (Health Economics Unit). 2010. *Bangladesh National Health Accounts 1997–2007*. Dhaka: Ministry of Health and Family Welfare.

HLSP/Mott MacDonald Ltd. 2010. *Bangladesh Health Sector Profile*. Dhaka: World Bank, Government of Bangladesh, and World Health Organization.

Hossain, A. M. Z., and I. Hussain. 2009. "Study on HRD in Bangladesh as a Prelude to the HRH Master Plan 2010–2040." Dhaka: JICA and Ministry of Health and Family Welfare, Government of Bangladesh.

Kaufmann, D., A. Kraay, and M. Mastruzzi. 2010. "The Worldwide Governance Indicators: Methodology and Analytical Issues." Policy Research Working Paper 5430, World Bank, Washington, DC.

MIS-DGHS (Management Information System-Directorate General of Health Services). 2009. *Health Bulletin 2008*. Dhaka: Ministry of Health and Family Welfare.

———. 2010. *Health Bulletin 2010*. Dhaka: Ministry of Health and Family Welfare.

Naripokkho. 2006. *Government Policies on Maternal Health in Bangladesh and the Impact on the Right to Health: Human Rights Impact Assessment (HRIA) Case Study*. Dhaka: Naripokkho.

Ostrom, E., L. Schroeder, and S. Wynne. 1993. *Institutional Incentives and Sustainable Development: Infrastructure Policies in Perspective*. Boulder, CO: Westview Press.

Ostrom, V., C. M. Tiebout, and R. Warren. 1961. "The Organization of Government in Metropolitan Areas: A Theoretical Inquiry." *American Political Science Review* 55: 831–42.

Peters, D., and R. Kayne. 2003. *Bangladesh Health Labor Market Study: Final Report*. Dhaka: Canadian International Development Agency.

SIDA (Swedish International Development Cooperation Agency). 2009. *Reality Check Bangladesh 2008: Listening to the Poor People's Realities about Primary Healthcare and Primary Education*. Dhaka: Edita Communications.

UPHCP (Urban Primary Health Care Project). 2010. "Second Urban Primary Health Care Project (UPHCP-II)." http://www.uphcp.org/index.php/welcome/home_body_more.

World Health Organization (WHO). 2006a. *The World Health Report 2006: Working Together for Health*. Geneva. http://www.who.int/whosis/mort/profiles/mort_searo_bgd_bangladesh.pdf.

———. 2006b. "World Mortality Country Factsheet 2006: Bangladesh." Geneva.

———. 2007. *Everybody's Business: Strengthening Health Systems to Improve Health Outcomes: WHO's Framework for Action*. Geneva. http://www.who.int/healthsystems/strategy/everybodys_business.pdf.

———. 2009. *World Health Statistics 2009*. Geneva.

———. 2010. *Health Systems: Governance*. http://www.who.int/healthsystems/topics/stewardship/en/index.html.

WHO BD (World Health Organization, Country Office for Bangladesh). 2010. "Noncommunicable Disease & Mental Health: Surveillance, Prevention and Management." WHO and Country Office for Bangladesh, Dhaka.

WHO SEARO (World Health Organization, Regional Office for South East Asia). 2007. "Capacity for Noncommunicable Disease Prevention and Control in Countries of the South-East Asia Region: Results of a 2006–2007 Survey." World Health Organization, Regional Office for South East Asia, New Delhi.

CHAPTER 4

National NCD Activities and Challenges

Orientation of the Public Sector

The public sector is oriented to primary health care with a focus on mothers and children as well as communicable disease interventions to meet the health-related Millennium Development Goals (MDGs). In terms of policy on noncommunicable diseases (NCDs), Bangladesh Health, Population and Nutrition Sector Development Programme (HPNSDP) 2011–16 has identified four NCDs—cardiovascular diseases (CVDs), cancer, diabetes mellitus, and arsenicosis—as major public health problems. The current Strategic Plan for 2011–16 has seven priority activities (drivers) of which one specific strategy is to expand NCD control efforts at all levels by streamlining referral systems and strengthening hospital accreditation and management systems (Government of Bangladesh 2011a). It recommends that the public sector focus on prevention and that investment in intensive care units and tertiary care be left to the private sector. Publicly financed insurance and health vouchers are proposed for protection of the poor against the costs of emergency care and catastrophic illnesses associated with NCDs. Although this approach was adopted in the sector program in 2004, implementation has been minimal, owing particularly to political uncertainty, even with the development of comprehensive plans of action.

While a good awareness-raising strategy is essential to keep policy makers abreast of present concerns, Bangladesh has no such system to achieve dynamic and responsive support from them (see box 4.1). However, the following strategies and guidelines on NCDs exist in Bangladesh (the first three with technical assistance from World Health Organization (WHO) Bangladesh):

- Strategic Plan for Surveillance and Prevention of Non-Communicable Diseases in Bangladesh 2011–15—Directorate General of Health Services (DGHS);
- National Cancer Control Strategy and Plan of Action 2009–15—DGHS;
- National Strategic Plan of Action for Tobacco Control 2007–10—National Tobacco Control Cell of the Ministry of Health and Family Welfare (MOHFW);

Box 4.1 Chapter Four Summary

- Public health is focused on mothers and children through primary health care and on communicable diseases, not NCDs.
- Primary health care has little public infrastructure to support NCD prevention and management. NCD program-based infrastructure is largely at tertiary level.
- Four NCDs—CVDs, cancer, diabetes mellitus, and arsenicosis—are seen as major public health problems in HPNSDP 2011–2016. The control of NCDs is one of its five priority areas.
- The Strategic Plan and the Program Implementation Plan for HPNSDP emphasize reducing morbidity and premature mortality from NCDs through actions at all levels and in an integrated manner.
- Several challenges stand out: strengthening the regulatory framework; harmonizing strategic planning and coordination across sectors; aligning the objectives and interventions in the HPNSDP Strategic Plan with the operational plans; refocusing the health system on prevention and away from treatment; tackling fragmented health service delivery; and filling NCD data gaps.
- Coordination is minimal among NCD stakeholders. The government should study how to use its resources to incorporate NCD prevention and treatment in public health.

- Guidelines for care of Type 2 Diabetes Mellitus in Bangladesh—Bangladesh Institute of Research and Rehabilitation in Diabetes, Endocrine and Metabolic Disorders (BIRDEM) Clinical Research Group;
- Injury Prevention Strategy and Action Plan for Bangladesh 2011–2020—DGHS (with technical assistance from WHO and United Nations Children's Fund [UNICEF]); and
- National Strategy on Disaster Health Management—DGHS.

There is little public infrastructure at primary health care level to support NCD prevention and management. NCD program-based infrastructure exists largely at tertiary level. There is a long tradition of specialty hospitals and foundations, public and nonpublic, dating back to the 1950s (see chapter 3), which provide preventive and curative care for NCDs, such as the National Institute of Diseases of Chest & Hospital (NIDCH) and BIRDEM. The overwhelming majority of these institutions are in Dhaka, although several, like BIRDEM, have affiliated institutions in districts around the country. Others, like National Heart Foundation Hospital and Research Institute (NHFH&RI), hold camps or specialty clinics in various locations. Several of these institutions are home to postgraduate medical specialty education in NCDs (see appendix 2).

The Strategic Plan and the Program Implementation Plan for HPNSDP emphasize the reduction of morbidity and premature mortality due to NCDs through actions at all levels and in an integrated manner, from primary prevention to treatment and rehabilitation during 2011–16. The operational plans under HPNSDP aim to strengthen health service delivery for effective management and referral; promote healthy lifestyles and practices; and develop a sound public health surveillance system to address the growing burden of NCDs.

The upshot is that a multitiered health system for chronic disease management has developed: the rich travel abroad to receive care, the middle class travel to India whenever possible or to private institutions, and the poor receive very few resources.

Country Activities

Although a comprehensive NCD prevention and treatment program has yet to be introduced into the primary tier of public health services, a number of activities, many of which are in the pre-action phase, are taking place in Bangladesh's health sector. The country activities on NCDs follow from the capacity described in chapter 3 through a variety of specialty hospitals and foundations, and active participation from public sector research foundations such as the National Institute of Population Research and Training (NIPORT) and the Institute of Epidemiology, Disease Control and Research (IEDCR), which play a leading role in national surveillance efforts.

The control of NCDs is one of five priority areas in HPNSDP. However, efforts to include NCD prevention and care have been less of a priority in light of the attention given to achieving the MDGs and the Health for All initiative focusing on primary care.

The government's approval and launch of the Strategic Plan for Surveillance and Prevention of Noncommunicable Diseases in Bangladesh 2007–10, and its update in 2011, have helped the country to make great strides toward addressing NCD surveillance and management by the health sector (box 4.2) (DGHS 2011).

Eight Areas of NCD Activities

The following is a brief overview of NCD activities, public and private.

Under the DGHS, the line director for Non-Communicable Disease Control (NCDC) is responsible for carrying out the government's NCD initiative in the health sector. However, outside the arsenic program (see just below), the major activities under this operational plan have been limited to conducting training for health care providers at different levels, organizing awareness-building workshops, and supporting selected hospitals/institutes like NHFH&RI, Ahsania Mission Cancer Hospital, and the Bangabandhu Sheikh Mujib Medical University through buying equipment (DGHS 2007). Outside NCDC, the Essential Services Delivery line directorate also provides limited NCD-related services at primary level: during the first year of HPNSDP implementation, it introduced mental health services, and trained nurses and pharmacists for identifying, counseling, and treating mental illness. Also, a National NCD Prevention Cell has been established at the DGHS for coordinating different NCD prevention and management activities.

Box 4.2 Strategic Plan for Surveillance and Prevention of NCDs in Bangladesh, 2011–15

The strategy has eight objectives:

- To raise the priority accorded to NCDs in development work at national level and integrate prevention and control of such diseases across all government departments.
- To establish an integrated mechanism of sustainable collection, analysis, and dissemination of essential data on NCDs and their major risk factors, and provide an evidence base for public health decision making for containing NCDs.
- To establish and strengthen national policies and plans to increase the capacity of the health system for prevention and control of NCDs.
- To promote interventions that strengthen health-promotion measures, including risk reduction and behavioral change through healthy lifestyle and well-being campaigns to combat public health threats caused by tobacco use, unhealthy lifestyle, physical inactivity, harmful use of alcohol, occupation- and environment-related diseases, mental illness, and injuries.
- To promote research for prevention and control of NCDs.
- To assist communities in terms of knowledge and creating a favorable environment to empower people to become responsible for their health.
- To develop a common platform by promoting network formation among the relevant stakeholders for surveillance, prevention, and management of NCDs so that they can participate in a regional network for prevention and control of NCDs.
- To monitor NCDs and their determinants and evaluate progress at the national level.

In 2007, the MOHFW introduced the Upazila NCD Project to develop NCD capacity among public and private providers in the project sites. Through this project, the DGHS expanded NCD health care delivery to district hospitals and, on a pilot basis, to three selected *upazila* health complexes by creating new posts for NCD specialists. By 2010, 782 physicians, 1,345 nurses, 1,451 medical technologists, and 1,347 health assistants had been trained under the project (Bleich *et al.* 2010). Based on the experience and results from the pilot, the model was replicated in 137 *upazila*s in fiscal year 2011/12. The model will be rolled out in other *upazila*s later. The project objective and activities include training of health care providers on awareness creation; establishing NCD corners with one medical officer and two nurses; equipping *upazila* health complexes with an electrocardiogram machine, glucometer, blood pressure machine, and weight–height scales; and referring to higher facilities for effective management of major NCDs.

Under HPNSDP, the NCD line directorate conducted training for 95,160 health care professionals including doctors, nurses, paramedics, and field workers (of both the DGHS and DGFP [Directorate General of Family Planning]) on major NCDs including identification and management of arsenicosis and violence against women. The line directorate also conducted workshops for community mobilization on NCDs for 175,500 community leaders, including local government members and religious leaders.

After 2006, the Centre for Injury Prevention and Research, Bangladesh (CIPRB), with the NCD line directorate, UNICEF, and the Alliance of Safe Children (TASC), maintained a community-based surveillance and prevention program titled Prevention of Child Injuries through Social Intervention and Education (PRECISE). The surveillance area covers around 200,000 people in three *upazilas* and provides comprehensive information on child injury in a rural setting (MIS-DGHS 2010). With the help of UNICEF and CIPRB, a road traffic accident and injury prevention model was piloted in three *upazilas* in 2006 and replicated in 101 *upazilas* by 2012. Under this model, health care providers are trained in injury prevention and mass awareness creation. The DGHS has been implementing the Decade of Action for Road Safety 2011–20 with the ministries of Communication, Local Government, and Home Affairs. To ensure effective collaboration of injury data and disaster management, a national crisis management center has been established at the DGHS.

Under the National Policy for Arsenic Mitigation 2004, several activities were implemented including community awareness; capacity building; a two-year (2008–09) house-to-house search to identify arsenicosis patients; a specialized arsenicosis management program; awareness raising of alternate sources of water; research and development; and efforts to coordinate the work of the public and nongovermental oragnization sectors. This arsenic mitigation program takes up the lion's share of the total budget for the NCD line directorate (Government of Bangladesh 2011b; MIS-DGHS 2010).

Since 1956, the Diabetic Association of Bangladesh (BADAS) has provided diabetic care as a nonprofit voluntary socio-medical service organization. An institute of BADAS, BIRDEM provides diagnostic as well as primary and secondary clinical care of diabetes (outpatient and inpatient). It also conducts the largest number of postgraduate courses in the private sector. BADAS has expanded its activities to cardiac care through its Ibrahim Cardiac Hospital & Research Institute to prevent and treat cardiac diseases, to create awareness, and to develop skilled human resources. With the Government of Bangladesh, the Netherlands Development Finance Company, and a consortium of local banks, BADAS is piloting the Health Care Development Program, which includes a 250-bed teaching hospital, 10 urban health centers in and around Dhaka, a 200-bed regional hospital in Sirajganj, 30–75 bed subregional hospitals (in Bogra, Pabna, Dinajpur, and Thakurgaon), and four peripheral health centers linked to the subregional hospitals. The aim of the program is to test a model of integrated care service delivery in urban and rural areas, with a focus on the major NCDs (BADAS 2011; Bleich *et al.* 2010).

With technical assistance from WHO, the public sector's effort on tobacco control includes enacting the Smoking and Tobacco Product Usage (Control) Act 2005, which restricted smoking in public places and tobacco advertising in publications and other mass media. It also mandated health-warning labels on tobacco products and arranged loans for farmers to switch from growing tobacco to other crops. Under this initiative, the Global Tobacco Surveillance System has conducted a Global Youth Tobacco Survey (in 2004 and 2007), a Global

School Personnel Survey (2007), a Global Health Professions Students Survey (2009), and a Global Adult Tobacco Survey (2009) with technical support from WHO and the Centers for Disease Control and Prevention (WHO BD 2009).

The Centre for Control of Chronic Diseases in Bangladesh aims to bring scientific rigor to studying the burden of disease (BOD) for NCDs, to develop community-based prevention and management programs, to evaluate the link between NCDs and poverty in Bangladesh, and to assess the health system's response to NCDs. The Centre is a collaboration between International Centre for Diarrhoeal Disease Research, Bangladesh (ICDDR,B), Bangladesh Rural Advancement Committee (BRAC), the Johns Hopkins Bloomberg School of Public Health, and the Institute for Development Studies. The Centre, begun in June 2009 as a five-year project, is funded by the U.S. National Institutes of Health National Heart, Lung and Blood Institute and United Health Group, and is part of a network of centers of excellence within a global chronic disease initiative in low- and middle-income countries. Further, the Centre aims to work closely with key stakeholders for NCDs in Bangladesh to translate globally synthesized and locally realized evidence into policy.

Since 2007, the Bangladesh Network for Non-Communicable Disease Surveillance and Prevention (BanNet) has served as a platform for collaborating organizations that promote and collect information on NCD surveillance in Bangladesh (19 institutions include the MOHFW, Bureau of Health Education, and specialty hospitals and foundations). The Alliance for Community-based Surveillance has been formed by some members of BanNet to lead the community-based surveillance and periodic population-based surveys on NCDs and their risk factors (DGHS 2007).

Challenges

The review of health systems and national NCD activities reveals several challenges to be overcome.

Strengthening the Regulatory Framework

Improving the regulations that govern the prevention and control of NCDs and their enforcement is critical. For example, the Smoking and Tobacco Product Usage (Control) act 2005 went into effect in May 2006, but surveys capturing the impact of the Act on tobacco use have yet to be conducted. An evaluation of implementation of the measures in the act is advisable so that revisions can be made to ensure maximum impact: the most popular brand of cigarettes is taxed at 67 percent, which is still below what is recommended (WHO 2010). Nor do health-warning labels meet minimum requirements for impact. Further, the ban on advertising of tobacco products under the act is incomplete as there are advertisements at the point of sale, via the Internet and as promotional offerings. Smoking is still permitted in designated smoking areas, indoor offices, restaurants, and public transport. Most important, the National Tobacco Control Cell is understaffed and underfunded.

Tackling Noncommunicable Diseases in Bangladesh • http://dx.doi.org/10.1596/978-0-8213-9920-0

Harmonizing Strategic Planning and Coordination across Sectors

Several NCD interventions exist in public and private sectors with very little national coordination. There has been no overall assessment of activities by different stakeholders to ensure synergies across these programs, and the focus of the MOHFW on NCDs remains limited to implementing NCD interventions through the NCDC operational plan and financing tertiary health facilities. The final evaluation of the Health, Nutrition and Population Sector Program (2003–11) noted that NCD operational plans were inadequate in leadership, programs, and implementation despite the priority attached to NCDs in the revised program implementation plan in 2008 (Government of Bangladesh 2011c). Also, coordination across sectors was weak. For example, there was no provision for linking key national interventions (for example, tuberculosis and the tobacco control program) that could yield a more robust impact on the NCD burden. The government should use its resources to take a leadership role and incorporate NCD prevention and treatment in the public health sector, supported by WHO and already involved nonprofit organizations, such as BIRDEM and NHFH&RI.

Aligning the Objectives and Interventions in the HPNSDP Strategic Plan with the Operational Plans

The NCDC operational plan, for example, focuses on awareness building, but has not fully pursued training activities of health care providers and strengthening prevention, detection, and management of major NCDs and/or risk factors within the primary health care system. Also, while the Bangladesh Health Workforce Strategy 2008 recognized the importance of continuous monitoring, of careful choices between the population's health needs and reality, and of evidence drawn from health research for preventing rising rates of NCDs, it has set neither a specific strategic goal to deal with the workforce to manage NCDs nor any activity for implementing the strategic objectives.

Equally, the Essential Services Package and the essential drugs list in the public sector do not have guidelines and products to meet the needs of the growing number of individuals at risk for and managing chronic conditions.

Refocusing the Health Service Delivery System on Prevention and Away from Treatment

NCDs are tackled at secondary and tertiary levels mainly through treatment in specialized facilities. Less emphasis is given to prevention at primary care level and to readily available low-cost treatment. Much of the investment in infrastructure and medical equipment in the specialized facilities could be saved if NCD prevention interventions were scaled up. For example, the DGHS should transition from preplanning to action in piloting an NCD program in the *upazilas*. Technical assistance is available from numerous nongovernmental agencies. This engagement should be intensified and a proposal for specific strategies developed so these can be incorporated into the sector's budget. Ideally, the *upazila* pilot project should be carefully designed so that it does not deplete nor diminish health sector resources, but in such a way that the intervention can be sustained in the pilot area and then scaled up to other *upazila*s.

Tackling Fragmented Health Service Delivery and Improving Coordinated Care

In addressing the MDG challenges, the health service delivery system—as in most developing countries—was structured to deal with "episodes" of maternal and child health illnesses and communicable diseases. Such fragmentation has led to lack of coordinated care that is critical for effectively managing NCDs. Shifting the BOD toward NCDs would require an integrated approach that ensures continuity of care.

Filling NCD Data Gaps

The Demographic and Health Surveys (conducted under the MOHFW as part of the worldwide Demographic and Health Survey program) focus on fertility, family planning, and maternal and child health. Their failure to include NCDs (apart from tobacco use) is an enormous missed opportunity to capture health behaviors and self-reported morbidity. They could be expanded to capture exercise, fruit consumption, salt intake, alcohol consumption, and more. Further, women should be included in the questions about tobacco consumption, to judge if there is a rise in smoking as income levels increase so that interventions can be targeted. The 2006 Bangladesh Urban Health Survey (NIPORT *et al.* 2008) captures many of these factors and could serve as a model.

Another important gap surrounds the National Risk Factor Surveillance, technically supported by WHO, which was completed in 2010 with preliminary results made available in August 2011. The detailed first-round findings must be used to inform the development of policy and followed by action in support of mitigating or reducing risk factor exposure among the population. Further, the surveillance must be routine. At present, there is no plan to conduct surveillance of morbidity and/or mortality due to NCDs. This information would benefit health sector planning and inform global understanding of the changing BOD.

In light of rapid urbanization, it has become more important that there be a uniform reporting system linking urban health care services to the DGHS-MIS. The MIS needs to present the picture for the entire country, both of NCDs and other important health indicators. The unique risks to the more than 35 percent of slum dwellers in urban areas must be captured so that services can be developed to meet the health needs of this disenfranchised population.

Many NCD issues have been well studied in South Asians generally, and Bangladeshis particularly, in the diaspora. It is possible that much can be learned from health and community-based interventions in those populations, particularly the urban populations, who may have similar health and disease patterns as the urban, higher-income in-country Bangladeshis. A systematic review of this literature (much generated by the National Health Service of the United Kingdom and by the National Institutes of Health in the United States) would serve to quickly inform decision makers and practitioners of its applicability and lessons learned.

References

BADAS (Diabetic Association of Bangladesh). 2011. "DAB: The Beginning of a Journey, Which Goes On." http://www.dab-bd.org/about_dab/history.html.

Bleich, S. N., T. L. P. Koehlmoos, M. Rashid, D. H. Peters, and G. Anderson. 2010. "Noncommunicable Chronic Disease in Bangladesh: Overview of Existing Programs and Priorities Going Forward." *Health Policy*. doi:10.1016/j.healthpol.2010.09.004.

DGHS (Directorate General of Health Services), MOHFW (Ministry of Health and Family Welfare). 2007. *Strategic Plan for Surveillance and Prevention of Non-Communicable Diseases in Bangladesh 2007–2010*. Dhaka: DGHS, MOHFW.

———. 2011. *Strategic Plan for Surveillance and Prevention of Non-Communicable Diseases in Bangladesh 2011–2015*. Dhaka: MOHFW.

Government of Bangladesh. 2011a. *Strategic Plan for Health, Population and Nutrition Sector Development Program 2011–16*. Dhaka: MOHFW.

———. 2011b. *Health Population and Nutrition Sector Development Program 2011–16: Program Implementation Plan*. Vol. 1. Dhaka: MOHFW.

———. 2011c. *Final Report On End-Line Evaluation of Health, Nutrition and Population Sector Programme*. Dhaka: Ministry of Planning.

MIS-DGHS (Management Information System-Directorate General of Health Services). 2010. *Health Bulletin 2010*. Dhaka: MOHFW.

NIPORT, MEASURE Evaluation, ICDDR,B and ACPR (National Institute of Population Research and Training; MEASURE Evaluation, International Centre for Diarrhoeal Disease Research, Bangladesh; and Associates for Community and Population Research). 2008. *2006 Bangladesh Urban Health Survey*. Dhaka: NIPORT, ICDDR,B, ACPR; Chapel Hill, NC: MEASURE Evaluation.

WHO (World Health Organization). 2010. *WHO Report on the Global Tobacco Epidemic, 2009: Implementing Smoke-Free Environments*. Tobacco Free Initiative (TFI). Geneva, Switzerland: WHO. http://www.who.int/tobacco/mpower/2009/en/index.html.

WHO BD (World Health Organization, Country Office for Bangladesh). 2009. *Global Adult Tobacco Survey: Bangladesh Country Report 2009*. Dhaka. http://www.who.int/tobacco/surveillance/global_adult_tobacco_survey_bangladesh_report_2009.pdf.

CHAPTER 5

Key Policy Options and Strategic Priorities

A Policy Options Framework for noncommunicable diseases (NCDs), developed by Engelgau *et al.* (2011), is practical and can be adapted for each country to develop and organize policy interventions based on its NCD program's stage of development and its management capacity (table 5.1). The framework is organized to address both population- and individual-based policy interventions (see box 5.1). Each intervention mobilizes different parts of the health and non-health sectors and requires very different inputs in terms of infrastructure, capacity, and skill sets, while yielding very different outputs and outcomes. Harmonizing both sets of policy interventions is necessary to ensure that the mix is right and that population-based policy interventions complement those delivered to individuals within the clinical care system.

Since each country is at a different stage of NCD program development, the framework integrates the four stages of the basic program management cycle: Assess, Plan, Develop/Implement, and Evaluate (appendix 3). Hence, the policy options for a country will depend on its stage of program development, its burden of disease (BOD), and its health system's capacity to tackle NCDs (Englegau *et al.* 2011). From a public policy perspective, the functions of *Assessment* and *Planning* are the inherent responsibility of government, mainly the Ministry of Health and Family Welfare (MOHFW), to lead (with input from key stakeholders) as part of its stewardship and regulatory roles. This is not to forget public and private health institutions, which may undertake these functions at their levels. The functions of *Implementation* and *Evaluation* will then be undertaken by different sectors and institutions. Policy options and strategies related to the stewardship and regulatory role of the government are represented by the MOHFW.

Without being prescriptive, the Policy Options Framework forms the basis for policy dialog, including how to integrate five global priority interventions to curb NCDs—as given in an article in *The Lancet* (Beaglehole *et al.* 2011)—into the national NCD program. The study had reviewed global and country

Box 5.1 Chapter Five Summary

- A Policy Options Framework for NCDs, using population- and individual-based interventions, is proposed.
- It works through five main areas: stewardship and regulatory policy; population-based interventions in both the non-health and health sectors; and individual clinical interventions for both prevention and treatment.
- Five key interventions to prevent and control NCDs globally are integrated in the policy framework and include tobacco control, salt reduction, improved diets and physical activity, reduction in hazardous alcohol intake, and essential drugs and technologies.
- The government should consider the strategic priorities in the context of reducing both poverty and upward pressure on public finance. In setting them, it should be selective and consider mainly the most prevalent NCDs (CVDs, cancer, respiratory infections, injuries, and diabetes) and their risk factors (high blood pressure, high tobacco use, unhealthy diet and nutrition, malnutrition and low birth weight, arsenic in water sources, air pollution, lack of physical activity, and alcohol consumption and substance abuse).
- The MOHFW will play the leading role in developing and implementing these strategic priorities and in forging, with other sectors, a multisectoral alliance to ensure synergy among the different actions.

efforts to prevent and control NCDs. The five interventions were based on existing evidence and several selection criteria including health outcomes, cost-effectiveness, low costs of implementation, and political and financial feasibility of scaling up. They are tobacco control, salt reduction, improved diets and physical activity, reduction in hazardous alcohol intake, and essential drugs and technologies. They require five overarching priority actions: leadership, prevention, treatment, international cooperation, and monitoring and accountability.

The policy options and strategies for Bangladesh, subsequently detailed in this chapter, draw on the Policy Options Framework (table 5.1) and on the five priority interventions, as well as the information given in the previous chapters on BOD, risk factors, system capacity, and national programs for NCDs.

Stewardship and Regulatory Policy Options and Strategies

The MOHFW, representing the health sector, has the leading role in combating NCDs, including mobilizing the non-health sector. Leadership is a key factor in improving health services and was the first overarching priority action identified by the Lancet NCD Action Group and the NCD Alliance for responding to the NCD crisis (Beaglehole *et al.* 2011; Peters *et al.* 2009).

In its Bangladesh Health, Population and Nutrition Sector Development Programme (HPNSDP) 2011–16 Strategic Plan, the MOHFW has identified various actions with the priority of "establishing a national center for NCDs as an umbrella organization for NCD alliance." The plan does not provide much detail

Table 5.1 Policy Options Framework for Prevention and Control of NCDs in Bangladesh

Population-based interventions		Individual-based interventions	
Non-health sector (National alliance for NCDs)	*Health sector (MOHFW)*	*Prevention (clinical) (MOHFW)*	*Treatment (public and private sector)*
Stewardship and regulatory policy options and strategies (Leading role for the MOHFW)			
• Assessing NCD mortality, morbidity, BOD, risk factors, and high-risk populations as well as NCD risk factor determinants in the non-health sector. • Assessing the gaps in the policy and regulatory framework for NCD prevention and control. • Assessing current and future public health spending and health system capacity (institutional and management capacity and system intelligence) as well as health service delivery capacity (facilities, human resources, drugs, and so on) and current utilization of ambulatory and inpatient care. • Reviewing evidence-based public policies, population-based interventions, and cost-effective prevention and treatment interventions (including in other similar countries). • Developing a national policy and multisectoral strategic plan for the prevention and treatment of NCDs in consultation with the major stakeholders (health and non-health, public and private). • Improving coordination across NCD programs in different sectors.			
Population-based policy options and strategies for the non-health sector (Role of multisectors)	Population-based policy options and strategies for the health sector (Leading role for the MOHFW)	Policy options and strategies for clinical prevention services (Leading role for the MOHFW)	Policy options and strategies for treatment services (Partnership role between public and private health sectors)
• Developing and enforcing laws and regulatory mechanisms for the non-health sector • Developing institutional and human capacity • Mobilizing the necessary financial resources • Developing an effective system for monitoring the results and for impact evaluation	• Strengthening health promotion and risk reduction interventions in the health sector for the general population and/or high-risk groups • Developing the institutional and human capacity to address NCD risk factor determinants and to manage population-based health promotion and risk reduction in the MOHFW • Developing an effective system intelligence and information technology for NCDs, and strengthen and expand the national surveillance system to include NCDs and their risk factors	• Developing and implementing basic health services for reducing risk factors and preventing NCDs in public health facilities • Strengthening the institutional and human resources capacity to provide facility-based health promotion, behavior change, and risk-reduction services • Mobilizing additional financial resources for the health sector and considering budget reallocation within the health sector in support of NCD prevention and treatment • Establishing a monitoring system for NCD prevention indicators in public health facilities and conducting impact evaluation studies	• Strengthening health service delivery to provide high-quality and effective NCD control and treatment services in selected public health facilities • Developing strategic purchasing mechanisms to motivate public and private service providers to provide cost-effective and quality prevention and treatment services • Developing and monitoring indicators related to NCD treatment including conducting impact evaluation studies

Source: Modified from Engelgau *et al.* 2011.

Note: MOHFW = Ministry of Health and Family Welfare; NCD = noncommunicable disease; BOD = burden of disease.

on the composition and scope of the proposed organization. However, if well established with broad representation from different sectors and public and private institutions involved in the management and control of NCDs, it may provide the required national leadership.

The following details the key stewardship and regulatory policies and strategies for the prevention and control of NCDs.

- *Periodically assess NCD mortality, morbidity, BOD, risk factors, and high-risk populations as well as NCD risk factor determinants in the non-health sector.* This report has documented what is known to date. However, assessments will need to be updated periodically using data from the Bangladesh Demographic and Health Survey, Utilization of Essential Service Delivery Survey, Bangladesh Urban Health Survey, national Management Information System (MIS), and other surveys, which should be further expanded to include modules related to NCD morbidity. Opportunities should be considered to expand and supplement ongoing surveys to meet the assessment needs for NCDs. In addition, other important areas will need assessment: the MOHFW will need to track utilization, expenditure, institutionalization of activities, and the "bounds" of surveillance—that is, the limits on what surveillance can do and what will need special studies.

- *Assess the gaps in the policy and regulatory framework for NCD prevention and control.* This assessment should cover tobacco, commerce, agriculture, trade, the environment (indoor and outdoor air), and the built environment in urban areas. Bringing new partners from the non-health sector of the government (agriculture, transport, urban planning, and finance) as well as private partners to develop policy and implement regulations to promote healthy lifestyles and prevent NCDs will be vital. For example, tobacco taxation by the finance sector, low carbon emission from industries by the commerce and industry sector, and regulating smoke emission from vehicles by the transport sector will have a substantial impact on the national NCD burden. Moreover, comprehensive provision of occupational health services for the well-being of workers in the nonformal sectors involving farming, road transport, mining, quarrying, and so on will be key to reducing injuries and other occupational NCDs. The *Common Framework for Action* of the NCD Strategic Plan 2011–15 had the following actions: review of existing laws and acts related to NCD control and prevention; and enactment, amendment, and enforcement of laws and regulations related to NCDs (DGHS, MOHFW 2011). Both actions are critical and need to be pursued.

- *Assess current and future public health spending and health system capacity (institutional and management capacity and system intelligence) as well as health service delivery capacity (facilities, human resources, drugs, and so on) and current utilization of ambulatory and inpatient care.* This assessment is critical for overall health strategy development and sector planning in achieving the health goals and improving health outcomes—not only for NCDs, but for all conditions. A full assessment would cover all health system components including governance, regulatory framework, and institutional capacity; health financing including current and future public health spending and out-of-pocket spending; and health service delivery and its infrastructure at all levels as well as its utilization, human resources (numbers and skills), pharmaceuticals and medical technologies, and health system intelligence. Such an assessment should be carried out periodically and use available surveillance and survey data, as from Bangladesh Health Facility Surveys. Special studies may be also needed.

The HPNSDP 2011–16 Strategic Plan includes an assessment of health system capacity and its components. The plan also developed strategies and interventions for all programs, including the prevention and management of NCDs. Its priority interventions to improve NCD services in the plan include: (a) strengthening behavior change communication activities for prevention of NCDs; (b) diagnosing and managing kidney diseases, diabetes, and arsenicosis patients in primary, secondary, and tertiary health facilities; (c) strengthening prevention awareness and diagnosis of cardiovascular diseases CVDs in all three tiers of facilities and treatment in secondary and tertiary levels; (d) screening for early detection of cancer and strengthening diagnosis and management including palliative care of cancer patients in secondary and tertiary hospitals; (e) implementing the strategic action plan on injury prevention, NCD, and tobacco control; and (f) updating and implementing the National Eye Care Plan as well as strengthening and expanding the Emergency Medical Services.

However, the NCD interventions spread across several operational plans under HPNSDP 2011–16 did not take into consideration this assessment, and some of the proposed priority interventions were not included, including (d) and (f) just above.

- *Review evidence-based public policies, population-based interventions, and cost-effective prevention and treatment interventions (including those in comparable countries).* The MOHFW has a primary role in reviewing evidence-based public policies in the non-health sector, risk reduction studies, and population-based interventions, as well as available studies on cost-effective prevention interventions and low-cost treatment protocols in comparable low-income countries. It should adapt those relevant to the country's context and capacity.

  There is ample evidence from international experience about cost-effective interventions such as tobacco control (particularly tobacco taxation), salt reduction, improved diets and physical activity, reduction in hazardous alcohol intake, enforcement of seat belt use, early detection/screening for high blood pressure/hypertension and diabetes, prescription of low-dose aspirin for high-risk CVD patients, and essential drugs and technologies (Beaglehole *et al.* 2011; Jamison *et al.* 2006). Table 5.2 provides an estimated cost of a package of interventions that would greatly reduce the risk factors and BOD of NCDs in three countries, which might inform choices for Bangladesh.

Table 5.2 Estimated Cost of Interventions to Reduce NCD Risk Factors in Three Countries

		Cost per person per year ($)		
	Interventions	China	India	Russian Federation
1. Tobacco use	Accelerated implementation of the WHO Framework Convention on Tobacco Control	0.14	0.16	0.49
2. Dietary salt	Mass media campaign and voluntary action by food industry to reduce consumption	0.05	0.06	0.16
3. Obesity, unhealthy diet, and physical inactivity	Mass media campaigns, food taxes, subsidies, labeling, and marketing restrictions	0.43	0.35	1.18
4. Harmful alcohol intake	Tax increases, advertising bans, and restricted access	0.07	0.05	0.52
5. Cardiovascular risk reduction	Combination of drugs for individuals at high risk of NCDs	1.02	0.90	1.73
Total cost per person		1.72	1.52	4.08

Source: Beaglehole *et al.* 2011.
Note: WHO = World Health Organization; NCDs = noncommunicable diseases.

With a low level of public health expenditure in Bangladesh of about $7.80 per capita, priority should be given to population-based interventions given their relatively low cost and greater population benefits. The use of traditional and mass media to send positive health messages about healthy diet, tobacco and drug use, optimal mental health, and so on, particularly to young people, would be another cost-effective intervention.

In terms of population-based interventions specifically, Asaria *et al.* (2007) modeled the effects of a reduction in salt intake by 15 percent and a key set of tobacco measures contained in the World Health Organization (WHO) Framework Convention on Tobacco Control (increases in the price of tobacco; enforcement of smoke-free workplaces; packaging and labeling changes; public awareness campaigns; and a comprehensive ban on advertising, promotion, and sponsorship) in 23 low- and middle-income countries, including Bangladesh, over 10 years (2006–15) (table 5.3).

In the area of clinical interventions, whether for prevention or treatment, it will be more effective for the MOHFW to collaborate with medical schools and research centers in Bangladesh. The MOHFW, with help from public or nongovernment research institutes, should explore cost-effective NCD screening programs at the community level with a special emphasis on CVDs and/or diabetes. The medical schools should update protocols to ensure provision of optimal NCD care in health facilities. Multidisciplinary research committees should be established in collaboration with academia and professional organizations to look into three areas: a sustainable funding mechanism for NCD research; networking of government agencies, nongovernmental organizations (NGOs), and the academic community to support research; and translation of research findings into action.

- *Develop a national policy and* multisectoral *strategic plan for the prevention and treatment of NCDs in consultation with the major stakeholders (health and non-health, public and private).* The health sector has a leading role in responding to

Table 5.3 Effects of Salt-Intake Reduction and Tobacco Control Interventions in Bangladesh, 2006–15

Type of intervention	Male	Female
Tobacco control (%)		
Increase in real price of tobacco products required to reduce smoking prevalence by 10%	24.7	24.7
Predicted decrease in smoking prevalence as a result of nonprice interventions	12.9	11.7
Predicted decrease in smoking prevalence as a result of price and nonprice interventions combined	21.6	20.6
Salt-intake reduction		
Reduction in salt intake (grams per day) by age group		
30–44	2.0	1.8
45–59	2.0	1.7
60–69	2.0	1.7
70–79	2.0	1.7
80–100	2.0	1.7
Associated reduction in mean systolic blood pressure by 2015 (mm Hg) by age group		
30–44	1.3	1.1
45–59	1.7	1.6
60–69	2.3	2.2
70–79	2.8	2.8
80–100	3.5	3.5

Source: Asaria *et al.* 2007.

NCDs, but many other government sectors, including finance, agriculture, foreign affairs, trade, justice, education, urban design, and transport, have to be part of the whole-of-government response, along with civil society and the private sector (Beaglehole *et al.* 2011). Although the MOHFW has a strategic plan for 2011–16 for managing NCDs, Bangladesh does not have a comprehensive national policy and multisectoral strategic plan for NCDs.

Such a plan should be developed urgently, given the rising NCD epidemic, involving several sectors (table 5.4).

- *Improve coordination across NCD programs in different sectors.* Several programs support different NCD programs but have little national coordination. The MOHFW will need to take a more active role in convening and facilitating the implementation of these programs to build on the successful ones and ensuring synergies across these programs. An overall assessment of current activities and efforts both in the public and private sectors will be an essential first step toward developing a national coordination mechanism.

Population-Based Policy Options and Strategies for the Non-Health Sector

- *Develop and enforce laws and regulatory mechanisms for the non-health sector.* Policy actions include:
  - *Strengthen tobacco control policies:* Reasonable progress has been made with a national tobacco policy. However, tobacco use is still high among both adults and children. Expanding on the core activities in the WHO Framework Convention on Tobacco Control is needed. The National Tobacco Control

Table 5.4 Role of the Different Sectors in the Prevention and Control of NCDs

Sector	Interventions
Finance	• Subsidies to encourage healthy food production • Increasing prices for tobacco and alcohol • Removal of subsidies for products harmful to health, such as tobacco leaf and tobacco products
Agriculture, food industry	• Production and marketing of healthy food, with a focus on "storage and processing" aspects of seasonal fruits and vegetables adapted to the local realities • Salt reduction in (semi)-processed food; reduction of transfat in food • Maintaining adequate land for agriculture and food systems; crop substitution for tobacco leaves • Monitoring and adequately regulating the growing agro-processing sector that is increasingly producing ready-to-eat and ready-to-cook food and fruit-flavored drinks for domestic consumption
AND	• Stricter environment standards (for example, on waste management and carbon emission) and enforcement should be practiced. Globally, a quarter of all preventable illnesses (for example, cancer, chronic obstructive pulmonary disease) are the result of poor environmental conditions where people live • Real estate developers can be encouraged or mandated to include physical exercise facilities in their projects • Access to clean energy
Infrastructure, transportation	• Optimal planning for road, transport, and housing to reduce environmentally costly emissions and traffic injuries and to improve accessibility to health services • Better transport, including cycling and walking opportunities, building safer and more livable communities, and accessible facilities for physical activities
Education	• Physical activity programs for schoolchildren • School food and nutrition programs • Production of an adequate number of health professionals with needed skills for NCD prevention and care
Social protection	• Improved coverage of NCD-related preventive and curative services at the primary health care level • Exemption of NCD patients from copayment for selected preventive and curative services
Legislation and law enforcement	• Development and enforcement of pro-health policies and regulations on drunk driving, home violence, and a smoke-free environment • Enforcement of air pollution legislation
Media	• Promotion of change in social norms concerning smoking, being sedentary, and alcohol abuse and advocating healthy lifestyles
Private sector	• Occupational health and work safety • Workplace wellness programs

Source: Adapted from Adelaide Statement on Health in All Policies, WHO, Government of South Australia, Adelaide, 2010, cited in World Bank 2011, 14.
Note: NCD = noncommunicable disease.

Cell has to be strengthened further to play the pivotal role in tobacco control activities.

To this effect, the government should consider developing a tax framework that includes all major tobacco products, which may have a great impact on reducing consumption. It is suggested that a price increase of 33 percent of tobacco products will be effective in reducing smoking (Engelgau *et al.* 2011). However, this should be carefully devised to take into account its impact on public finance in terms of tax revenues, on agriculture in terms of production, and on labor in regard to job losses (Engelgau *et al.* 2011). For the national budget for FY2011/12, the finance minister proposed (in a measure that was passed) to increase supplementary duty on all brands of cigarettes by 2 percentage points (over the current rate) and to increase prices at varying rates—more in case of cheaper brands—and to increase supplementary duty on chewing tobacco from the current 20 to 30 percent (Government of Bangladesh 2011). The Government of Bangladesh may benefit from the experience of the Philippines in the successful introduction of the sin tax (box 5.2).

The government may also consider strict implementation of other non-price policy interventions already in place such as banning tobacco-product advertisements and banning smoking in government premises and public places (including transport) as a starting point to further expand the ban to larger public areas, as well as pushing through tobacco supply reductions and information dissemination. Global efforts in strengthening tobacco control policies are ongoing and tapping into these may prove useful.

- *Strengthen food regulation policies:* Evidence-based interventions exist in many countries. For example, legislation requiring the food industry to substitute 2 percent of transfat with polyunsaturated fat, at $0.50 per adult, is a primary intervention for the prevention of heart disease. Similarly, legislation to regulate the production and importation of food products with reduced salt content will have great benefits in reducing high blood pressure, stroke, and heart disease. Alternatively, a voluntary reformulation of the most consumed food products by the food industry in Bangladesh may be pursued through dialogue with industry leaders. Studies show that a salt reduction strategy is highly cost effective (see table 5.3). The MOHFW should lead a massive public health campaign for reducing salt content in the diet as processed food intake is not that high among the population and most of the salt is added during cooking. However, there is growing availability of processed food from both national and international food industries, which would require legislative and voluntary measures by the industry. The experience of Argentina in reaching agreements with the food industry and various companies on a progressive and voluntary course to reduce salt in processed foods provides a practical example (Daniel 2011).
- *Strengthen control policies related to road traffic injuries:* Road traffic injuries represent an increasing burden of morbidity and mortality. Improving road conditions is critical but will need large infrastructure investments and will only come into effect over the long term. Over a shorter time frame, however, law enforcement for the use of seat belts and helmets, coupled with a behavior-change campaign, would be feasible and effective policy measures to reduce the burden of road traffic accidents.
- *Strategies to reduce child injury:* Beyond infancy, injury is the leading cause of death among children in Bangladesh. To prevent childhood injuries and premature deaths, such as those due to drowning or road traffic accidents, strategies would include separate components for home (for instance, parents' and caretakers' awareness building through mass media, educative entertainment, and interpersonal communication), school (such as a grade-specific safety curriculum that covers safety risks, injury-prevention

Box 5.2 "Sin Tax" Reform in the Philippines

The Philippines is Southeast Asia's top tobacco-smoking country. Smoking does not just cause cancer and lung diseases. It is the leading cause of stroke and heart attack resulting in about 50,000 deaths per year. In fact, it causes more stroke and heart attacks than diabetes, hypertension, obesity, and high cholesterol combined (according to the 2008 National Nutrition and Health Survey).

Until very recently, the country had some of the lowest cigarette taxes and prices in the world and the strongest tobacco lobby in Asia, notably, vested interests powerfully represented in the legislature, as exemplified in the excise tax system that protected profits of established domestic alcohol and tobacco firms against new market entrants and foreign firms (rates on imported products, for example, were almost 225 percent as high as the highest applied to domestic products).

A new Tobacco and Alcohol Excise Tax (Sin Tax) Law was ratified by the bicameral Philippine Congress in December 2012. Its purpose was threefold:

- *To reduce the harm on the population of tobacco (and alcohol)*—tobacco smoking is the number one preventable risk factor for premature death. It is expected that the tax will cut the number of cigarette packs consumed each year from 5.0 billion to less than 2.5 billion.
- *To simplify the current excise tax system* on alcohol and tobacco products and fix long-standing, structural weaknesses, including no linking of the excise tax to retail price inflation (tobacco excise collection had declined from 0.50 percent of gross domestic product (GDP) in 1997 to 0.25 percent in 2010).
- *To generate revenues* to finance a Universal Health Care Program under the National Health Insurance Program (which would receive 80 percent of the incremental revenues from the new tax) and the medical assistance and health enhancement facilities program (20 percent), after deducting the support from the tax allocated for tobacco farmers' livelihoods. It will also reduce the smoking-related economic burden of 177 billion pesos in 2011 (around $4.4 billion at early 2013 exchange rates), including health care costs, productivity losses, and premature death losses. This burden dwarfs revenues from tobacco excise taxes.

The law sharply raises the average excise tax rate on cigarettes' retail prices from 29.1 percent in 2012 to 52.5 percent in 2013 (and to 63.0 percent by 2017, which adheres to WHO's Framework Convention on Tobacco Control). It also brings in annual excise tax indexation from 2018. In the first year (the 2013 budget year), the government is expected to raise additional revenues of 23.4 billion pesos from cigarettes.

The following were the key success factors in getting the legislation passed:

- *Framing the tax reform as a "health measure".* There was broad-based political support for universal health care—and politicians do not want to be seen as against health. This was the ultimate response to critics of sin tax reform.
- *Political support and coalition building.* Having political support at the highest levels was the most important factor. President Aquino, elected in 2010, gave his unwavering backing, as did the new chairs of the powerful Ways and Means Committees in Congress (the previous

box continues next page

Box 5.2 "Sin Tax" Reform in the Philippines *(continued)*

chairs opposed the measure). Opposition from tobacco-farmers' groups was softened by an allocation of some of the incremental revenues of the excise tax. An alliance between the tobacco and alcohol industries was forestalled by concessions to the alcohol lobby in the bill laid before the lower house to obtain the swing vote from the Nationalist People's Coalition. And many traditional (nonreform) politicians were won over by the promise of a portion of the incremental revenues for universal health care going to their congressional districts.

- *Effective strategic communication.* Directed to people on the street, communication stressed how reform would benefit people's health and how sin tax reform could save more lives.
- *Evidence-based research and scenario modeling.* Analytical support came from academe as well as the Asian Development Bank, International Monetary Fund, WHO, and the World Bank, which generally spoke with one development partner voice.

Source: Authors, based on information compiled from presentations made by Jeremias Paul, Jr, Undersecretary, Department of Finance, the Philippines; Kai Kaiser, Senior Economist; and Roberto Iglesias, Senior Health Specialist, the World Bank, at the Human Development Learning Week, February 2013, at the World Bank, Washington, DC.

---

procedures, and basic first aid), and the community (for example, community crèches for children aged 1–5 years, and swimming lessons for children of 4–10 years). Moreover, mother and child health clinics can start with awareness building among parents and caregivers of children during their regular service contacts for prenatal checkups and immunizations, and so on.

- *Develop the institutional and human capacity of the non-health sector to address NCD risk factor determinants.* Developing the regulatory framework will be ineffective unless coupled with that of the institutional capacity to implement these regulations and programs. For the non-health sector, capacity development will be needed in several areas to enact and implement these policies, such as the adoption of an economically sound tax policy for tobacco control and its effective implementation; the alignment of incentives toward NCD prevention in the sale and consumption of food with high salt and unhealthy fats; and the implementation of occupational health services to prevent occupational injuries in the informal sector.

- *Mobilize the necessary financial resources to support NCD prevention and control in the non-health sector.* An effective strategy would require engaging leadership outside the health sector by increasing awareness about the economic impact and financial burden on each of the affected sectors as well as the cost-effectiveness of the proposed interventions. Professional organizations and civil society can play an important role. These actions could be supported by allocations of some of the revenues from the tobacco tax (and possibly alcohol tax) to the sectors involved in NCD prevention and control.

- *Develop an effective system for monitoring the results of implementing the population-based interventions and evaluating their impact in the non-health sector.* Monitoring the results and evaluating the impact of these policies will be key for building the evidence base for future policies as well as to ensure that resources are being used effectively in order to sustain the support of the non-health sector.

Population-Based Policy Options and Strategies for the Health Sector

• *Strengthen the health promotion and risk reduction interventions of the MOHFW for the general population and/or high-risk groups.* The MOHFW should strengthen its health promotion, behavior change, and risk reduction programs to include promoting healthy lifestyles, and increasing awareness about risks of smoking, obesity, and injury risk from respiratory tract infections. These measures should form the cornerstone of the ministry's strategy. If there are no effective risk reduction interventions, as the age of the population increases, people will become increasingly sick and consume an ever-larger proportion of the national health care budget.

However, the burden of lifetime illness may be compressed into a shorter period before death, if the age of onset of the first chronic illness can be postponed, mainly through risk reduction interventions. This "compression of morbidity" has been observed in many places such as the United States, Canada, and the European Union, where people not only live longer but their quality of life is improved by the reduction of sickness disability at the end of life (Fries 2005).

Given the progression of disability-adjusted life years (DALYs) in Bangladesh, it appears that the increase in the number of healthy life years is not quite in line with the increase in life expectancy, mainly due to NCDs. Available resources for promotion and risk reduction should therefore be better mobilized, used, and harmonized. Several programs have a component for promotion and behavior change, which need to be consolidated across different programs to be more effective. For example, the Arsenic Control Program is large and commands many resources, which can be used more effectively in more strategic areas like screening and early detection of hypertension and diabetes. Also, increased health literacy has been reported to be effective in promoting healthy lifestyles (Yajima *et al.* 2001). Community-wide campaigns and point-of-decision prompts (that is, signs placed by elevators and escalators) are effective in reducing NCD risk factors (ECOSOC 2010). Such interventions can be undertaken with the private sector. National and multinational companies in Bangladesh may have corporate social responsibility programs that support community development and public-good interventions that can be mobilized to support a national NCD literacy campaign.

• *Develop the institutional and human capacity to manage population-based health promotion and risk reduction in the MOHFW.* Developing the regulatory framework will not be effective unless coupled with the development of the institutional capacity to implement these regulations and programs. In the health sector, the MOHFW will need to develop the skills of its staff in designing and implementing behavior-change campaigns and health literacy programs to promote healthy lifestyles. In addition, sensitization of the population to the use of allopathic medicine and its benefits is needed as part of preventive services.

- *Develop effective system intelligence and information technology for NCDs, and strengthen and expand the national surveillance system to include NCDs and their risk factors.* Several pilot studies and interventions have been implemented and need to be evaluated. Developing effective system intelligence that will collect NCD morbidity and mortality data from the service delivery system, monitor trends in risk factors, analyze epidemiological data, and triangulate data from different sources is becoming increasingly crucial. This will be especially true for tobacco and injury policies. Interventions may include using electronic records to track care utilization, analyzing electronic police reports to track road traffic accidents, monitoring unhealthy food content (salt, sugar, fat, monosodium glutamate, caffeine, and artificial flavors) in processed food, and restricting sale of unhealthy food in places like schools and amusement parks.

  Much has already been done toward a national surveillance system. The national risk factor survey under way needs to be institutionalized and adequately resourced with staff and equipment. Moreover, an integrated strategy for injury surveillance is needed. Public and private institutions should be tapped and coordinated in support of NCD surveillance efforts. In addition, enhanced morbidity and mortality surveillance in BanNet and Matlab are critical for building national capacity.

Policy Options and Strategies for Individual Clinical Interventions for the Prevention of NCDs in the Health Sector

- *Develop and implement basic health services for reducing risk factors and preventing NCDs in public health facilities,* including the provision of lifestyle interventions to care seekers for improving self-regulatory behavior. Studies conducted in Bangladesh have demonstrated that diabetic education programs and lifestyle interventions of a nonpharmacological approach can significantly improve self-regulatory behavior, which in the long run can reduce morbidity and mortality related to diabetes (Hoque *et al.* 2009) and high blood pressure (Choudhury *et al.* 2010). A key cost-effective intervention for the prevention of heart attack and stroke is the use of the "polypill" containing aspirin, beta-blocker, thiazide diuretic, angiotensin-converting enzyme inhibitor, and statin (Jamison *et al.* 2006; Laxminarayan *et al.* 2006). This intervention costs less than $1 per person a year and is therefore feasible to introduce and scale up in public health facilities.

  The MOHFW will need to revise the Essential Services Package to include cost-effective preventive and risk reduction interventions to be implemented in the public health sector. Adequate human resources and infrastructure need to be put into place. These interventions may include screening for high blood pressure, cholesterol, and diabetes as well as an interpersonal communication program for smoking cessation and improved diet. Also, existing interventions for combating communicable diseases may be used to prevent and detect early specific NCDs, and may include, for example, expanding the scope of immunization programs to include human papillomavirus (which causes cervical cancer); strengthening maternal and child nutrition programs to ensure proper intrauterine growth; and collaborating with existing sexual and reproductive health programs to raise awareness of early signs of cervical and breast cancers among women (Marquez and Farrington 2012).

- *Strengthen the institutional and human resources capacity to provide facility-based health promotion, behavior change, and risk reduction services.* As indicated, the MOHFW will need to expand the Essential Services Package to include NCD-related interventions. In addition, there will be a need for commensurate efforts to strengthen the institutional and human resources capacity to provide these services, particularly those related to integrating primary health care (PHC) services (notably community clinics with secondary and tertiary levels) and to ensure continuity of care. That would include training of service providers, infrastructure, clinical quality assessment, and provider guidelines. To facilitate this process, it is important to develop a list of the optimal level of services to be delivered at various levels of care for the prevention of NCDs and the management of selected NCDs (such as heart disease) depending on the level of resources available in the public sector.

  Given the impact of climate change on health and NCDs—especially the psycho-social aspect and mental health issues—the MOHFW initiative, through the Climate Change and Health Promotion Unit, should be integrated with the proposed national center for NCDs (see *Stewardship and Regulatory Policy Options and Strategies* above) for better coordination.

- *Mobilize additional financial resources for the health sector and consider budget reallocation within the health sector in support of NCD prevention and treatment.* The public health sector is underfinanced and has limited fiscal space to allocate additional resources to priority health programs, including NCDs. The MOHFW will need to engage in a constructive dialogue with the Ministry of Finance and the Prime Minister's Office to mobilize additional resources for the sector, while considering potential efficiency gains in the existing budget. If MOHFW increases the allocation of resources incrementally to its NCD programs, these investments in NCDs today will save future costs that the MOHFW, and ultimately the Ministry of Finance, will otherwise have to bear as a result of inaction.

- *Establish a monitoring system for NCD prevention indicators in public health facilities as well as conduct impact evaluation studies.* There are several starting points that can be implemented simultaneously and then expanded. For example, some process and output indicators may be included at the level of the NCD operational plan that are directly linked to the planned activities and commensurate with their level of funding. In parallel, basic NCD interventions (such as blood pressure and blood glucose measurement for screening, and health promotion) that are implemented in PHC health facilities up to the *upazila* level need to be monitored and included in routine reporting. In addition, data on critical NCD prevention interventions in tertiary hospitals that are already implemented should be collected.

  Similarly, several other operational plans such as Health Education and Promotion; Quality Assurance; and Information, Education and Communication can support some NCD prevention activities, such as promoting healthy lifestyles, tobacco awareness, tobacco cessation support, diet counseling (vegetables, salt, fats), and safe water use (free of arsenic), where their related indicators should be routinely collected. The scope of the health information system should be then gradually broadened to collect routine information on NCD prevalence, intervention, and quality of care from tertiary to primary health facilities.

Policy Options and Strategies for Individual Clinical Interventions for the Treatment of NCDs in the Health Sector

- *Strengthen health service delivery to provide high-quality and effective NCD control and treatment services in selected public health facilities.* Given the limited resources in the public sector, there may be limitations to providing the full range of NCD treatment in all public health facilities. However, the MOHFW can strengthen the treatment protocols for the management and control of the most critical NCDs in selected public health facilities in order to retool health service delivery for NCDs. To this effect, the physician and nonphysician workforce will need treatment guidelines, clinical protocols, service standards, knowledge, and skills to diagnose and treat NCDs within the primary care system. Best practices of NCD treatment may be piloted, and those evaluated and proven effective and appropriate for Bangladesh may be scaled up. In addition, adequate supply and access to essential medications are needed, especially for the poor. More important, collaboration with the private sector, NGOs, medical schools, and specialized centers may enhance provision of such services for wider segments of the population.

  Table 5.5 provides a list of suggested services for managing acute and chronic cases of stroke, coronary heart diseases, and diabetes, tailored to the different levels of health care in Bangladesh.

Table 5.5 Recommended Services at Various Levels of Care in the MOHFW in Bangladesh

Services	Stroke	Coronary heart diseases and diabetes
Primary health care (PHC) level (union subcenter and community clinic)		
Screening and diagnosis	• Identification of signs and symptoms of acute stroke, transient ischemic attack (TIA), ischemic heart disease • Screening for hypertension (HTN), diabetes mellitus (DM) (only urine test), dyslipidemia, and oral contraceptive pill use	• Noninvasive screening (history, tobacco use, overweight/obesity, family history of stroke/coronary artery disease, lifestyle) • Screening for HTN and management with simple drugs (treat all cases with >160/100mmHg BP)
Management acute/ emergency	• Basic of resuscitation • Refer immediately to a tertiary care center (*if not equipped to carry out acute management or in case of unstable/ deteriorating condition*)	• Oral nitrates • Aspirin
Chronic care	• Prescription for secondary prevention • Tobacco cessation for users	• Secondary prophylaxis for rheumatic heart disease • Tobacco cessation for users • Regular physical exercise • Dietary modification
Follow-up	• Lifestyle education, follow-up for compliance along with refill of medicines, referral of complicated cases, and rehabilitation	
Secondary health care level (upazila health complex, UHC)		
Screening and diagnosis	*Same as PHC level +* • Investigation: ECG, total cholesterol	*Same as PHC level +* • Investigations: ECG (for diagnosis of acute presentations like ACS, pulmonary embolism, T-wave changes for cerebral hemorrhage, electrolyte imbalance); and total cholesterol • Blood sugar level: follow algorithm for insulin sliding scale • Diagnose and treat gestational DM/DM with pregnancy • Diagnose and treat DM with HTN care
Management acute/ emergency	*Same as PHC level +* • Temperature maintenance	*Same as PHC level +* • Evaluate the hemodynamic status • Inpatient care for uncontrolled HTN • Treatment of CHD with aspirin/Clopidogrel, statin, beta blocker/ACE inhibitor • Acute management and immediate referral of diabetic emergency (hypoglycemia, ketosis, coma)
Chronic care	*Same as PHC level +* • Prescription of multiple drugs and anticoagulants	*Same as PHC level +* • Treatment of HTN, DM
Follow-up	• Lifestyle education, follow-up for compliance, investigations and change of prescriptions if needed, referral of complicated cases to a tertiary-level center, and rehabilitation	
District level		
Screening and diagnosis	*Same as UHC level +* • Additional investigations: pulse oximetry, ECHO, X-ray.	*Same as UHC level +* • Noninvasive screening: BMI, and waist circumference • Screening for HTN and DM • Investigations: ECG, X-ray, lipid profile, ECHO

table continues next page

Table 5.5 Recommended Services at Various Levels of Care in the MOHFW in Bangladesh *(continued)*

Services	Stroke	Coronary heart diseases and diabetes
Management acute/ emergency	• Inpatient care • Management of BP with parenteral agents • Supportive care • Prophylaxis for deep venous thrombosis • Acute rehabilitation • Refer to a tertiary care center in case of significant, pressure effects, or surgical candidates with hemorrhage	• Evaluate the hemodynamic status • Thrombolysis • Inpatient care for uncontrolled HTN with end-organ complications • Treatment of diabetic ketoacidosis in all facilities that have electrolyte management equipment
Chronic care	• Tobacco cessation for users • Prescription of multiple drugs and anticoagulants	• Tobacco cessation for users • Secondary prevention • Treatment of HTN, DM
Follow-up	• Lifestyle education, follow-up for compliance, investigations and change of prescriptions if needed, referral of complicated cases to a tertiary-level center, and rehabilitation	

Source: Adapted for the Bangladesh health sector from Prabhakaran and Ajay (2009) with inputs from Professor Dr. Shah Monir Hossain, former Director General of Health Services, MOHFW, Bangladesh; Prof. Dr. Md. Habibe Millat, Vice Chairman and Honorary Director, Bangladesh Medical Research Council, Bangladesh; and Assoc. Prof. Dr. Sohel Reza Choudhury, Project Coordinator—Anti Tobacco Program, Department of Epidemiology and Research, National Heart Foundation Hospital and Research Institute, Bangladesh.
Note: MOHFW = Ministry of Health and Family Welfare.

- *Develop strategic purchasing mechanisms to motivate public and private service providers to provide cost-effective and high-quality prevention and treatment services.* As indicated earlier, payment of service providers in Bangladesh is not linked to performance. In pursuing strategies to reduce the burden of NCDs, the MOHFW may explore, on a pilot basis, the benefits of linking payments to PHC providers to preventive services including NCDs. In the private sector, this can be initiated through private health insurance programs that cover employees of large private companies by aligning payments with provider performance in relation to reduction of NCD risk factors and prevention. Also, outsourcing expensive and high-tech clinical interventions to the private sector may be more cost effective than in the public sector, given the high cost of investment and maintenance of medical equipment.

- *Develop and monitor indicators related to NCD treatment including conducting impact evaluation studies.* Similar to the proposed actions related to monitoring of prevention activities, some process, output, and quality indicators related to clinical treatment of NCDs may be included in the relevant operational plans such as Essential Service Delivery and Improved Hospital Service Management as well as collected from those health facilities that provide these services. Such service delivery indicators may include number of detected cases (high blood pressure, hypercholesterolemia, and hyperglycemia), number of follow-up visits, number of treated/controlled cases, and case fatality rate.

Lead Role of the Ministry of Health and Family Welfare

Tackling NCDs in a comprehensive way would require developing a strong multisectoral program that combines both prevention and treatment interventions, as well as forging a partnership between the public and private sector.

The above policy options and strategies provide a menu for building this comprehensive program over the years.

A key initial challenge is to determine the strategic priorities that will constitute the building blocks in the short and medium term. Given the impoverishing effect of NCDs and their ever-increasing costs, the government should consider these priorities in the context of poverty reduction and reducing upward pressure on public finance. Operationally, it is important to capitalize on current activities and take into account available resources. In addition, these strategic priorities should be selective in terms of considering mainly the most common risk factors—namely high blood pressure, high tobacco use, unhealthy diet, malnutrition and low birth weight, and arsenic in water sources.

The MOHFW, for the health sector, will have the leading role in these strategic priorities, which will require full integration in the relevant operational plans. The MOHFW will also need new skills to work effectively with other sectors to build a multisectoral alliance to ensure synergy among the different actions.

References

Asaria, P., D. Chisholm, C. Mathers, M. Ezzati, and R. Beaglehole. 2007. "Chronic Disease Prevention: Health Effects and Financial Costs of Strategies to Reduce Salt Intake and Control Tobacco Use." *The Lancet* 370 (9604): 2044–53.

Beaglehole, R., R. Bonita, R. Horton, C. Adams, G. Alleyne, and P. Asaria. 2011. "Priority Actions for the Non-Communicable Disease Crisis." *The Lancet* 377 (9775): 1438–47.

Choudhury, K. N., R. S. Mahmud, M. Salehuddin, S. Zareen, S. N. Uddin, and S. K. Ghosh. 2010. "A Trial on the Effects of Life Style Interventions in High-Normal Blood Pressure." *Cardiovascular Journal* 2 (2): 195–203.

Daniel Ferrante, Nicolas Apro, Veronica Ferreira, Mario Virgolini, Valentina Aguilar, Miriam Sosa, Pablo Perel, and Juan Casas (2011). Feasibility of salt reduction in processed foods in Argentina. Rev Panam Salud Publica. 2011; 29(2): 69–75.

DGHS (Directorate General of Health Services), MOHFW (Ministry of Health and Family Welfare). 2011. *Strategic Plan for Surveillance and Prevention of Non-Communicable Diseases in Bangladesh 2011–2015.* Dhaka: MOHFW.

ECOSOC (United Nations Economic and Social Council). 2010. "Health Literacy and the Millennium Development Goals: United Nations Economic and Social Council (ECOSOC) Regional Meeting Background Paper (Abstracted)." *Journal of Health Communication* 15 (Suppl 2): 211–23.

Engelgau, M. M., S. El-Saharty, P. Kudesia, V. Rajan, S. Rosenhouse, and K. Okamoto. 2011. *Capitalizing on the Demographic Transition: Tackling Noncommunicable Diseases in South Asia.* Washington, DC: World Bank.

Fries, J. 2005. "The Compression of Morbidity." *The Milbank Quarterly* 83 (4): 801–23.

Government of Bangladesh. 2011. *Towards Building A Happy, Prosperous and Caring Bangladesh: Budget Speech 2011–12.* Dhaka: Ministry of Finance.

Hoque, M. A., M. S. Islam, M. A. M. Khan, R. Aziz, and H. A. M. N. Ahasan. 2009. "Achievement of Awareness in a Diabetic Population." *Journal of Medicine* 10 (Suppl 1): 7–10.

Jamison, D., J. Breman, A. Measham, G. Alleyne, M. Claeson, D. Evans, P. Jha, A. Mills, and P. Musgrove, eds. 2006. *Disease Control Priorities in Developing Countries*, Second Edition. Washington, DC: World Bank.

Laxminarayan, R., A. J. Mills, J. G. Breman, A. R. Measham, G. Alleyne, M. Claeson, P. Jha, P. Musgrove, J. Chow, S. Shahid-Salles, and D. T. Jamison. 2006. "Advancement of Global Health: Key Messages from the Disease Control Priorities Project." *The Lancet* 367 (9517): 1193–208.

Marquez, P., and J. Farrington. 2012. "Africa's Next Burden: Non-Infectious Disease." *British Medical Journal* 345: e5812.

Peters, D., S. El-Saharty, B. Siadat, K. Janovsky, and M. Vujicic. eds. 2009. *Improving Health Service Delivery in Developing Countries: From Evidence to Action*. Washington, DC: World Bank.

Prabhakaran, D., and V. Ajay. 2009. *Noncommunicable Disease in India: A Perspective*. Centre for Chronic Disease Control discussion report for the World Health Organization, New Delhi.

World Bank. 2011. *Toward a Healthy and Harmonious Life in China: Stemming the Rising Tide of Non-Communicable Diseases*. http://www.worldbank.org/content/dam/Worldbank/document/NCD_report_en.pdf.

Yajima, S., T. Takano, K. Nakamura, and M. Watanabe. 2001. "Effectiveness of a Community Leaders' Programme to Promote Healthy Lifestyles in Tokyo, Japan." *Health Promotion International* 16 (3): 235–43.

Leading Causes of Mortality and Disability-Adjusted Life Years and Risk Factors for Bangladesh, 2010 Estimates

Causes	Deaths (%)	DALYs (%)	Risk factor	DALYs (%)
Cardiovascular and circulatory diseases	15.9	6.3	Tobacco smoking	5.4
Neoplasms	13.7	7.3	Household air pollution	4.9
Chronic respiratory diseases	9.9	6.3	Dietary risks	4.8
Neonatal disorders	9.4	14.4	Occupational risks	4.4
Lower respiratory infections	7.0	4.6	High blood pressure	3.5
Neurological disorders	4.2	4.7	Iron deficiency	3.0
Tuberculosis	3.0	2.3	Childhood underweight	2.7
Digestive diseases (except cirrhosis)	2.9	1.4	High blood glucose	2.5
Diabetes mellitus	2.9	1.6	Particulate matter pollution	2.0
Other communicable, maternal, neonatal, and nutritional disorders	2.9	2.7	Suboptimal breastfeeding	1.4
Cirrhosis of the liver	2.7	1.5	Low physical activity	1.2
Drowning	2.5	2.6	Drug use	0.8
Chronic kidney diseases	2.3	1.6	High body-mass index	0.7
Other noncommunicable diseases	2.2	5.7	Intimate partner violence	0.7
Diarrheal diseases	2.0	2.6	Alcohol use	0.7
Self-harm and interpersonal violence	2.0	1.7		
Protein-energy malnutrition	1.7	1.4		
Urinary diseases and male infertility	1.7	1.0		
Falls	1.6	1.4		
Poisonings	1.3	1.2		
Transport injuries	0.8	1.4		

Sources: Institute for Health Metrics and Evaluation, forthcoming; Global Burden of Disease Study 2010; Bangladesh Results by Cause 1990–2010, Seattle, WA.
Note: Cause-specific mortality and morbidity estimates are age-standardized rates per 100,000 population. DALYs = disability-adjusted life years.

NCD Treatment, Research, and Training Institutions in Bangladesh

Facility	History	Size and staffing	What is provided	Provision of outreach to secondary and primary care
BIRDEM Diabetic Association of Bangladesh	Not-for-profit hospital founded in 1956. WHO Collaborating Center for research on prevention and control of diabetes since 1982	500-bed hospital	Comprehensive diabetic health care delivery through outdoor and indoor patient care facilities. Training of Primary Health Care physicians on diabetes National Health Network Diabetes awareness campaign Diabetes education for individual and family members Seminars, workshops, and conferences Young diabetic camps	Yes, affiliated institutions in 55 out of 64 districts
National Institute of Cardiovascular Disease	Established in 1978; public institution	79 doctors, 163 nurses, and 24 paramedics	**Emergency cardiac care** Treatment of chronic CVDs including angioplasty and stenting, surgical procedures for coronary, valvular, vascular, etc. **Modern diagnostic facility** Coronary angiography Imaging Electrophysiological study **Academic** Postgraduate courses on cardiology Training of nurses and paramedics on CVD **Dissemination** Seminars and workshops	N/A
National Institute of Traumatology and Orthopaedic Rehabilitation (NITOR)	Established in 1972; public institution	325-bed hospital, with 75 beds for casualty Outpatient and inpatient facilities	Traumatic and orthopedic services, with 24-hour emergency service, and limb and brace center	N/A
National Institute of Mental Health (NIMH)	Established in 1981; public institution	150-bed hospital Outpatient and inpatient facilities	Treatment and management of mental disorders. Research in mental health	N/A

table continues next page

Facility	History	Size and staffing	What is provided	Provision of outreach to secondary and primary care
National Heart Foundation Hospital & Research Institute (NHFH&RI)	Established in 1978 for prevention and control of CVDs in Bangladesh; autonomous institution	300-bed hospital	Provides modern diagnostic and therapeutic facilities for cardiovascular problems Conducts epidemiological research and therapeutic trials on CVD Publishes awareness building booklets and educational materials on prevention of CVDs Organizes heart camps at different places of the country to treat cardiac patients educate and motivate people about prevention and control of CVDs Arranges seminars and conferences on CVDs	Yes
National Institute of Diseases of Chest & Hospital (NIDCH)	Established in early 1950; public facility	600-bed hospital Outpatient and inpatient facilities for patients with chest diseases	**Clinical** Medical and surgical treatment for chest disease including chronic obstructive pulmonary disease Direct Observation Treatment Centre for TB treatment including Multi-drug Resistant Tuberculosis treatment **Academic** Postgraduate training on chest disease (medical and surgical) **National Asthma Centre**—an affiliated institution and specialized facility for treatment of asthma, allergic disorders, and COPD	N/A
National Institute of Cancer Research and Hospital	Established in late 1980s	50-bed hospital soon to be upgraded to 300 beds Outpatient and inpatient facilities	**Curative care of cancer patients** Detection Medical Surgical Radiological **Hospital-based cancer registry** **Community-based cancer registry** **Epidemiological research** Publishes Annual Report	N/A

table continues next page

Facility	History	Size and staffing	What is provided	Provision of outreach to secondary and primary care
Dhaka Ahsania Mission Cancer Hospital	Not-for-profit foundation providing low-cost, quality treatment, especially for the poor	N/A	**Modern diagnostic and management facilities for cancer** Follow up of cancer patients Hospital-based cancer registry **Major clinical services** Surgical oncology Medical oncology Radiotherapy Brachytherapy **Diagnostic services** Tumor markers a comprehensive array of Imaging technologies, endoscopy, colonoscopy, and bronchoscopy, etc. **Research in cancer epidemiology and treatment**	N/A
Bangabandhu Sheikh Mujib Medical University	Established in 1965 as postgraduate institute; converted to university in 1998	1,500-bed hospital with 36 departments and 4 faculties Outpatient and inpatient facilities	**Academic** Postgraduate training on cardiology, hematology, nephrology, oncology, etc. **Clinical** Medical and surgical treatment for different NCDs, including diagnostic facilities.	N/A
Tertiary-level specialized hospital and medical college (9 in total)	Established between 1946 (Dhaka) and 1970 (Rangpur); public facility	Different capacities Outpatient and inpatient facilities	**Academic** Graduate training on different areas **Clinical** Medical and surgical treatment for different NCDs	N/A
National Institute of Neurosciences and Hospital	Established in 2012; public facility	300-bed hospital Outpatient and inpatient facilities	Provides treatment and management for neurological disorders, including stroke, epilepsy, etc. 24-hour emergency services and diagnostic facility	N/A

table continues next page

Facility	History	Size and staffing	What is provided	Provision of outreach to secondary and primary care
Institute of Epidemiology, Disease Control and Research (IEDCR)	Established in 1962; public institution	115 staff in 7 departments	Research in behavioral and biochemical risk factors for major NCDs Runs a Behavioral Risk Factor Surveillance System	N/A
Centre for Control of Chronic Diseases in Bangladesh	Established in 2008; not-for-profit international organization		Conducted population-based study to assess NCD burden in 4 surveillance sites Conducts studies on NCDs risk factors in urban and rural Bangladesh	
Tertiary-level private medical college and hospitals (4 in total)	Established between 1953 (Holy Family Red Crescent MCH) and 2003 (Enam MCH); private institutions	Different capacities Outpatient and inpatient facilities	Conducts cardiac surgery and provides coronary care unit support including diagnostic services **Academic** Graduate medical training	
Tertiary-level specialized private hospitals (4 in total)	Established between 2004 (Lab Aid) and 2006 (Square Hospital and United Hospital); private, for-profit institutions	Different capacities Outpatient and inpatient facilities	Conducts cardiac surgery and provides coronary care unit support, including diagnostic services	
Nongovernmental organizations (5 in total)	Founded between 1992 (Zia Heart Foundation) and 2003 (Eminence); nongovernmental organizations	Different capacities	Conducts research activities, behavior change communication, advocacy, and healthcare services	

Source: Directorate General of Health Services, Ministry of Health and Family Welfare. 2012. *Super Brands of NCDs in Bangladesh.* Dhaka: Ministry of Health and Family Welfare.

Note: BIRDEM = Bangladesh Institute of Research and Rehabilitation in Diabetes; COPD = chronic obstructive pulmonary disease; CVD = cardiovascular diseases; NCD = noncommunicable disease; WHO = World Health Organization.

Assessment and the Program Management Cycle

In each program management stage of the framework, action areas that play an important role in both modes of interventions for prevention and control of noncommunicable diseases (NCDs) are identified. In each action area, there are options for both population-based and individual-based interventions. The population-based interventions are divided into policy options that lie within the control of the non-health and health sector. Similarly, the individual-based interventions are divided into preventive services at the clinical level and treatment options at the primary and secondary levels of care. Tertiary-level care options are not discussed in the framework, as the evidence on cost-effectiveness indicates that provision of financial protection to the poor against catastrophic expenditure is the main area where government should intervene.

In the policy context, both intervention modes are not always mutually exclusive. A number of areas on cross cutting include assessing system capacity, and developing national plans and strategies and human resources. Considering both modes is important and practical—although the balance depends on the situation.

The rationale and activities for each program management stage are as follows.

At the *Assess* stage, information is collected that will facilitate efficient and effective planning and preparation, and help strategically target actions and prevention and control efforts.

The *Plan* stage entails analyzing information collected from assessments, engaging key stakeholders for prevention from inside and outside the health sector (for example, transportation, agriculture, commerce, urban planners, and business leaders) for treatment among both public and private sectors. NCD stakeholders extend from government and ministries of health to private sector providers, from individuals to communities, nongovernmental organizations (NGOs), health care providers, academia, and donor partners. Consensus and ownership are all needed for plans to be widely advocated, adopted, financed, and eventually institutionalized.

The *Develop/Implement* stage is where broad implementation of prevention policies and scaling up of clinical interventions span all the health sector and, potentially, the non-health sector. Developed country experiences provide some grounding. However, major retooling, and in many cases innovation, will be needed to develop effective policies for both individual- and population-based health promotion in developing countries. Currently, in terms of clinical services, only a few care delivery models exist and their effectiveness remains unclear. Health services in facilities will need retooling; clinical quality assessment procedures need development and implementation; and drug policies need to assure quality, availability, and affordability of essential medications.

A major challenge in the *Develop/Implement* stage is human resources. But financing non-health and health sector population-based policies as well as resource-intensive clinical prevention and treatment services imposes a substantial cost burden on governments.

The importance of the *Evaluate* stage becomes clear when we understand that countries are currently spending substantial resources on NCDs, especially on individual-based treatment. As capacity rises, programs launch, and investments grow, evaluating progress at all levels is essential to assure that goals are reached. For NCDs, the track record is short, experience is limited, but some new initiatives have already been launched or are being planned. Decision makers will greatly benefit from evaluating progress and health systems performance as utilization patterns evolve in the future.

For some stages, such as *Assess* and *Plan*, the framework will produce country-level policy options and actions, as well as strategies, which will be similar for each country across the region. However, *Develop/Implement* and *Evaluate* will tend to be more country specific, depending on burden and capacity.

Some important elements may lie beyond the capacity of a country acting alone and are not feasible at the country level, such as efforts in comparative effectiveness assessments for new service delivery interventions, and a regional approach (multilateral) may be complementary to domestic effort.

Some other key points to be considered:

- Prevention policies are implemented by both the health sector and key areas of the non-health sector such as finance (tobacco tax) and transportation (injury prevention). By contrast, most treatment policies are implemented within the health sector.
- Prevention policies apply to the general public with spin-off applications in the private sector. Treatment policies apply equally to both public and private sectors.
- Financing for burden assessment and population-based prevention efforts are mostly publicly funded, while that for treatment is both public and private with most (currently) coming from private sources.

This assessment took a health systems approach to describe health system capacity in general, with a focus on elements that are important to NCDs. Rather than a comprehensive assessment, we focused on finding strengths that might be enhanced and deficits that could be addressed. For this approach, we adopted the *Health Systems Assessment Approach: A How-To Manual* from the United States Agency for International Development for our health sector capacity assessment. It covers governance, health financing, health service delivery, human resources, pharmaceutical management, and health information systems. We extensively reviewed the World Health Organization (WHO) NCD capacity tools used for global surveys in 2000 and 2005 and a new tool under development/implementation in 2009 and 2010 and adapted suitable components into our tool. All country-based consultants used the same assessment tool, which included both objective and descriptive measures of capacity.

Environmental Benefits Statement

The World Bank is committed to reducing its environmental footprint. In support of this commitment, the Office of the Publisher leverages electronic publishing options and print-on-demand technology, which is located in regional hubs worldwide. Together, these initiatives enable print runs to be lowered and shipping distances decreased, resulting in reduced paper consumption, chemical use, greenhouse gas emissions, and waste.

The Office of the Publisher follows the recommended standards for paper use set by the Green Press Initiative. Whenever possible, books are printed on 50% to 100% postconsumer recycled paper, and at least 50% of the fiber in our book paper is either unbleached or bleached using Totally Chlorine Free (TCF), Processed Chlorine Free (PCF), or Enhanced Elemental Chlorine Free (EECF) processes.

More information about the Bank's environmental philosophy can be found at http://crinfo.worldbank.org/crinfo/environmental_responsibility/index.html.

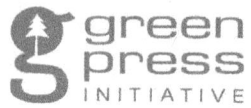